Mukhlisa Turopova

Practical Zoology: Invertebrate Forms and Functions

© Mukhlisa Turopova

Practical Zoology: Invertebrate Forms and Functions

By: Mukhlisa Turopova

Edition: December '2025

Publisher:

Taemeer Publications LLC (Michigan, USA / Hyderabad, India)

ISBN 978-93-6908-508-8

9 789369 085088

Book	:	Practical Zoology: Invertebrate Forms and Functions
Author	:	Mukhlisa Turopova
Publisher	:	Taemeer Publications
Year	:	'2025
Pages	:	74
Title Design	:	*Taemeer Web Design*

Instruction Safety rules in laboratories .

1. Until students become familiar with the "rules," frontal (where everyone does the same thing) and group work (where everyone does different types of experiments) are used. not to transfer.
2. Use only clean, dry and good tools during work. use.
3. Not tasting any substances, eating in laboratories not eating.
4. Do not give any substances from the laboratory room to anyone and do not allow students to take any substances or objects home at their own discretion.
5. Handle volatile substances with caution. smell
6. Do not lean over a container into which something is being poured (because small drops of liquid can splash into your eyes). possible).
7. Do not lean over a steaming porcelain dish (because the droplets and flying dry particles can burn the face). possible).
8. Eye protection (because even the smallest drop of a harmful substance can lead to loss of vision) comes).
9. When holding a test tube containing the liquid being heated, keep its mouth facing away from you and your friends (because if it is heated too much, the liquid will boil and splash onto the page). possible).
10. To heat solutions of substances in test tubes, add them to 1/3 of the test tube. casting
11. Store solids only in dry test tubes. heating
12. When heating glass containers, do not touch them to the wick of the alcohol lamp (because the wick will be cold and may crack and break the container). possible).
13. Thick-walled glass containers (jars, glasses, cylinders) and measuring cups, as well as porcelain mortars, should be heated in a flame. not to heat.
14. Light an alcohol lamp using only a match, but do not light it at an angle to a burning lamp (as spilled alcohol may ignite). possible). Extinguish the alcohol lamp with only the cap on. (don't blow).

1- Laboratory exercise

Subject : Common amoeba (Amoeba proteus), Arcella (Arcella vulgaris), Difflugia (Difflugia pyriformis) and The structure of foraminifera (Elphidiumcrispum), asexual and sexual increase.

Phylum: Sarcomastigophora Class : Sarcodidae, i.e. pseudopods – Sarcodina

Category: Amoebas- Amoebina, Amoebas with shells-Testacea

Representative: Simple amoeba-Amoeba proteus, Amoebas with shells- Arcella common

The purpose of the work: To study the structure, nutrition, and reproduction of representatives of the Sarcodidae class based on laboratory experiments, and to obtain complete information through conducting experiments.

Required equipment : plates depicting the structure and movement of amoebas, microscopes, stained micropreparations of amoebas, water with live amoebas, slides and coverslips, droppers, pieces of filter paper, water with amoebas, pieces of wax or plasticine.

Theoretical part : Unicellular animals are widespread in the seas, oceans, freshwater bodies and moist soil . There are also many species of them that live as parasites in humans, invertebrates and vertebrates . Although they are morphologically similar to individual cells of multicellular animals , they are physiologically independent organisms. Some parts of the cell cytoplasm are adapted to carry out vital functions , they are called organoids or organelles . is called.

in ponds and lakes among rotting plant debris (Figure 6). It feeds on algae and bacteria . Its size is 0.4-0.5 mm , and its body consists of cytoplasm. consists of.

It consists of two layers: a glassy clear and dark outer layer - ectoplasm, and an inner layer - endoplasm, which is relatively liquid, with a granular structure. The amoeba moves by forming pseudopods from its body . The pseudopods also perform the function of capturing food substances . This is the amoeba's nutrition by phagocytosis. The captured substance (food) passes into the cytoplasm along with water, and a digestive vacuole is formed around it. Under the influence of enzymes of the cytoplasm , food is digested in the vacuole , and residual substances are excreted from various parts of the amoeba's body as a result of the rupture of the digestive vacuole . is released.

The contractile vacuole performs the function of osmoregulation. Together with water, oxygen passes into the cytoplasm. Residual substances formed from the breakdown of proteins and carbohydrates, CO_2 Thus, the contractile vacuole is a part of the cell that performs the functions of division and respiration . are organs.

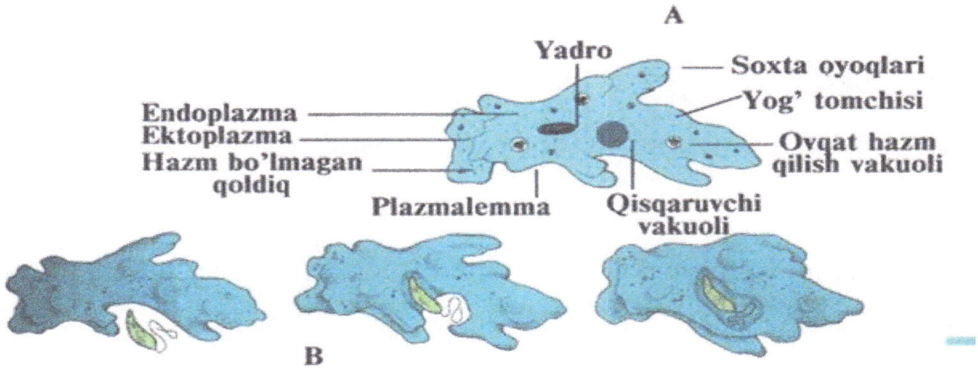

Figure 1. A- structure of amoeba, B- nutrition of amoeba (phagocytosis).

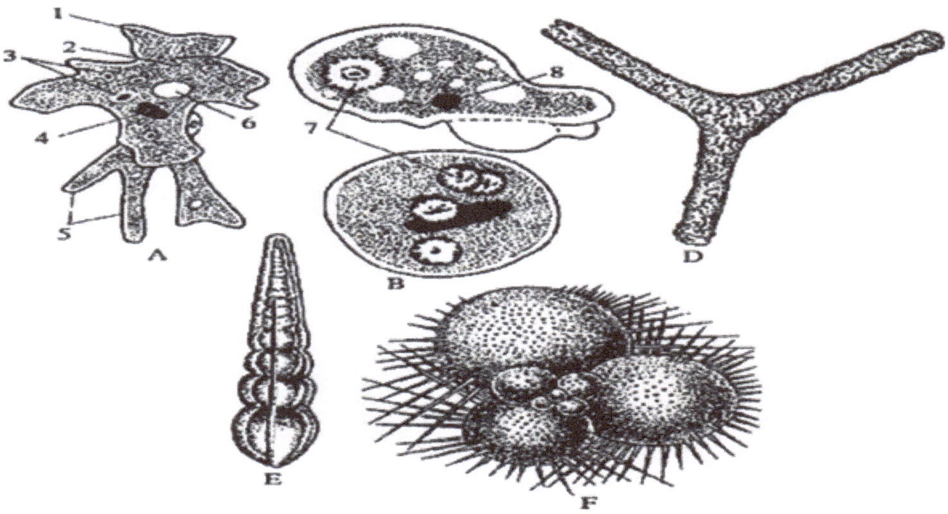

Figure 2 Pseudopods.

A - **simple amoeba, B - amoeba. D, E, F - various foraminifera (D - sand shell, E - calcareous shell with chambers arranged in a row, F - calcareous shell with chambers arranged in a spiral): 1 - ectoplasm, 2 - endoplasm,**

3 - digestive vacuoles, 4 - nucleus, 5 - pseudopods, 6 - contractile vacuole, 7 - nucleus divided within the cyst, 8 - encapsulated erythrocyte.

The nucleus is located in the endoplasm of the amoeba. However, it can only be observed in specially stained micropreparations. Amoeba reproduces asexually only by division.

It divides once every 1-2 days at 20-25 ^{0C} when there is enough food .

Work order:

1. **Work: To observe the structure and movement of amoeba,** a drop of amoebic fluid is taken with a pipette and placed on a glass slide , a coverslip is placed on it, then we place it in the microscope and leave it for a few minutes. The reason is that when the preparation is prepared, disturbed amoebae become rounded. At this time, it is impossible to see them . possible.

first look at the preparation with a small lens of a microscope . By adjusting the light falling on the preparation, we can see the external structure of the animal. If we look closely at the amoeba, we can see that it changes its shape and moves slowly. If we observe the amoeba for a long time, we can also see that it is catching food with the help of its false legs. possible.

Now we carefully turn the large objective of the microscope. Under the large objective, the outer and inner layers of the amoeba are visible. By changing the illumination intensity, it is possible to see the nucleus, vacuole, and other parts of the amoeba's body .

2. **work. Freshwater and water-shelled amoebas series** .

Arcella and difflugues can be found in ponds inhabited by amoebas or at the bottom of aquariums that have not been cleaned for a long time . Their bodies consist of cytoplasm, but are enclosed in a protective shell. The shell of the arcella is saucer-shaped and consists of a horn-like substance similar in composition to chitin. Its color is clear in young arcella , and as it grows , it can be light golden or brownish copper . There is one hole at the bottom of the shell, from which pseudopods protrude . Its protoplasm contains 2 nuclei and several contractile cells. will have vacuoles .

The shell of the Diffluga is pear-shaped with a narrower mouth. located.

The main part of the shell is formed by the liquid secreted by the cytoplasm. However, it may also contain sand particles and shells of brown algae . These particles first pass through the cytoplasm of the difluga and, after leaving it , stick together , forming shells of various shapes . Like amoebas, these also divide increases.

Work order.

1. To observe the movement of amoebas , a drop of water is placed on a glass slide and covered with a coverslip . It is observed through the small objective of the microscope, and after the amoeba is found , it is transferred to a large objective and its movement is studied. Pay attention to the false legs of the amoeba, which sometimes appear and sometimes disappear. Pictures depicting the gradual change in the shape of an amoeba Draw.

2. Observe one of the large amoebas through a microscope lens and distinguish between its ectoplasmic and endoplasmic layers, and identify the digestive and contractile vacuoles. find.

Note the decrease in the water content of the contractile vacuole. The nucleus of living amoebas is not visible, it can only be seen in specially prepared stained micropreparations. Draw a picture of the general appearance of an amoeba.

3. Place a drop of water from ponds or from the bottom of aquariums that have not been cleaned for a long time on a slide and cover it with a coverslip with wax or plasticine legs. Observe the preparation first through the small objective of the microscope and then through the large objective . Pay attention to the top and side views of the Arcella shell . Pictures of it in different forms Draw.

4. preparations using the above method , observe the shape and composition of the diffusion shell using different microscope lenses, and photograph it. Draw.

Assignments on the topic .

Draw a picture of the amoeba's feeding, movement, and structure in your notebook.

Review questions.

1. Characteristic features of the Sarcomastigophora type Tell me?
2. Structure and development of amoeba how?
3. Difference between a simple amoeba and a shell amoeba What's the difference?
4. Amoeba movement, nutrition, and defense how?
5. How to grow amoeba in the laboratory shall we check?

2- Laboratory exercise.

Topic: Phylum Chlorophyta, Class Volvocida, Structure of Volvox sp. (volvox), Representative of Colonial Fungi

Type. Sarcomastigophora Class. Mastigophora

Subclass. Phytomastigina Order. Phytomonads-Phytomonadina

Representative. Volvox-Volvox

The purpose of the training session: to study the structure of euglena and colonial hyenas and to get acquainted with their representatives.

Learning outcomes (student): will study the structure of euglena and colonial ciliates, become familiar with their various species, explain their structure, and gain an understanding of them.

Required materials and equipment: water sample with Volvox, water sample with colonial ciliates, microscopes, slides and coverslips, droppers, napkins, plates, filter papers, iodine solution.

The content of the work. Volvox is the largest (up to 2 mm) of the colonial anemones, and can be found in ponds, lakes, and sometimes in marshes. Volvox is a spherical, unicellular anemones that live in colonies.

Several thousand individuals (cells) in a colony are connected to each other by cytoplasmic bridges. The structure of each cell exactly

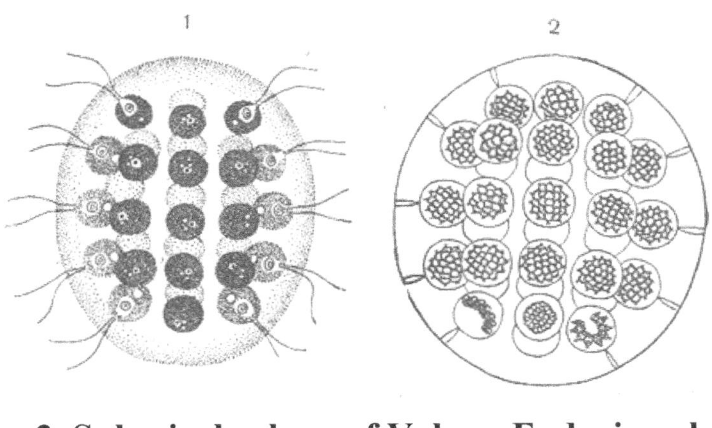

Figure 3. Spherical colony of Volvox-Eudorina elegans .

1-3-cell colony; 2-asexual reproduction.

It resembles the cell structure of Euglena, that is, each individual has two cilia, a nucleus, chromatophores, a contractile vacuole, and an "eye" (stigma).

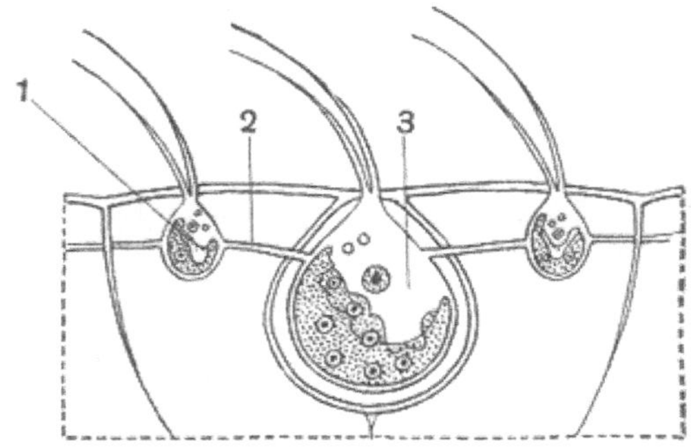

Figure 4. Part of a Volvox aureus colony.

1- vegetative cells of the colony; 2-cytoplasmic bridge; 3-the largest cells in the colony, as a result of their development, new daughter colonies are formed.

Therefore, each of the individuals in the volvox should be considered an independent unicellular organism. However, most of these individuals do not have the ability to divide and reproduce, they are called somatic cells in the volvox. There are very few individuals in the volvox that have the ability to reproduce, only 4-
There may be 10. These are parthenogonidia or "reproductive vegetative cells."

They do not have any organoids and serve only for reproduction. As a result of the division of these individuals (parthenogonia) in the colony into several, a new young colony is formed.

Therefore, within the Volvox (within the "mother") there are several young ("daughter") colonies.

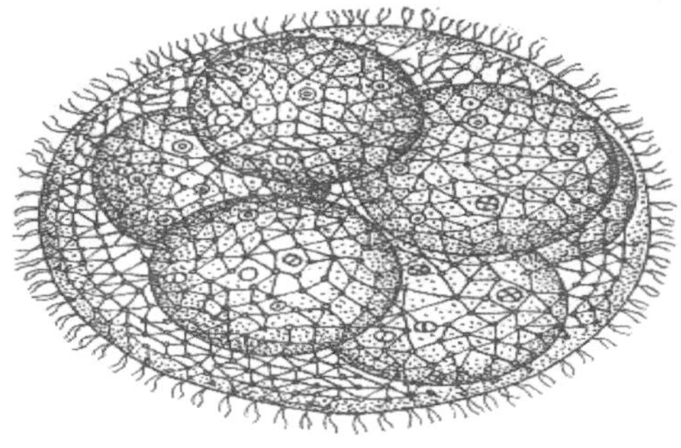

Figure 5. Young colonies within a Volvox-Volvox aureus mother colony.

Procedure: A drop of water samples containing Volvox and other colonial colonies is placed on a glass slide. First, it is observed under a small microscope objective. Attention is paid to the general shape of the colonies and their movement. Due to the oscillation of the colony's colonies, the ball always moves forward in a circular motion. Young colonies are found inside the Volvox body and their structure is observed. give it..

Assignments on the topic.

Draw a picture of a Volvox colony in your notebook.

Control questions :

1. What are the main representatives of the Khivchin people? 2. Formation, development and reproduction of Volvox how?

3. What are the similarities and differences between green euglena and volvox?

3- Laboratory exercise

Subject: The structure and function of the water strider Gregarina , a representative of the Apicomplexa or Sporozoa subphylum , Gregarinina class . development.

Type: Sporozoa

Class: Gregarines - Gregarinina

Category: True gregarines- Eugregarinida Representative: Gregarina - Gregarina

Objective : To gain information about representatives of the class Spores.
Studying the structure of gregarine based on laboratory experiments

Required equipment: Microscope, Gregarina plate, scalpel, tweezers, sharp-edged scissors, watch, specimen and coverslips, straightening needles, forceps, saline solution, ether, carmine or a live black mite (if black mite is not available, flour beetle larvae will do) , eyedropper, water.

Theoretical part : Gregarinas are the largest among spore-forming organisms (from 10 to 16 microns), parasitic in the intestines or body cavities of invertebrates (water fleas, mites, dragonflies, earthworms) -picture).

The body of gregarines consists of 3 parts: the anterior epimerite, the middle protomerite, and the posterior deutomerite.

The nucleus is located in the deuteromere. The epimerite part serves to attach to the inner cells of the cell.

Gregarines reproduce sexually . Gregarines do not have a "mouth" or "pharynx" contractile vacuoles. Therefore, the feeding, respiration, and excretion processes of gregarines are carried out based on osmotic pressure. Dividing the development cycle of gregarines into 3 stages possible;

1. Adulthood of gregarines reach.

2. The formation of gametes and fertilization (population) occur. 3. Zygotes (oocysts) develop and sporozoites are produced. to be.

The movements of gregarines vary . For example, the water gregarine moves like a rocket, then releases a clear liquid through pores in its abdomen.

Work order.

1. Several live black worms are placed in a glass and ether soaked in cotton wool is poured into it. When the worms stop moving , they are opened. To do this, the abdomen of the worm is cut with sharp scissors on both sides, up to the border of the head , and the shoulder part is separated with tweezers. The head and abdomen are fixed in the bath with clamps and water is poured over it. As a result, the internal organs float to the surface of the water. A transverse section is taken from the intestines of the worm, placed in a watch glass, and physiological saline is added with a dropper. solution is poured. Then rectifier needle using is captured. Harvest was is mixed with water, a drop of it is placed on a glass slide , covered with a cover glass , and observed through a small objective of a microscope . Since the gregarine is quite large, it is difficult to see the white spot on the surface of the water with the naked eye. possible .

1. To observe the movement of gregarine , a drop of carmine and a little bit of stone powder dissolved in water is added to the gregarine on the slide and the coverslip is closed. Then it is placed under a microscope for observation. Since the liquid is black, the fluid flowing out of the pores in the abdomen is well visible . it seems.

2. To observe the structure of the gregarine , a small pressure is applied to the coverslip using a straightening needle , stopping the movement of the gregarine. This allows us to clearly see the deuteromere and protomere parts, which have a rather large bubble-like nucleus , as well as the cuticle, clear ectoplasm, and granular, less clear endoplasm . possible.

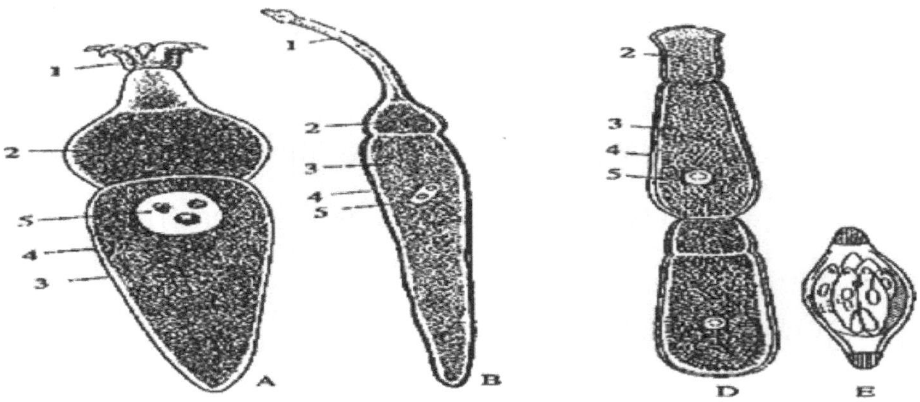

6 .Grtgarinas,

A - CoryceUa annata, V - Stylocephalus longicollis, D - **Gregarina blaLt&cutn, E - gregarina spore: 1 - epimerite, 2 - protamedt, 3 - deutomerite, 4 - cuticle, 5 - souvenir,**

Assignments on the topic.

1. the movement of Gregarina . Observe the traces left behind by Gregarina's movement . and Draw a picture .
2. the structure of the Gregarina and add its picture to the album. Draw.

Control questions:

1. Gregarina's structure?
2. How do Gregarina reproduce ? 3. Where do Gregarinas parasitize? 4. How do Gregarinas move? does?
5. What is the systematic position of Gregarina?

4- Laboratory training

Topic: The structure and function of the Infusoria (Paramecium caudatum), a representative of the Infusoria or Ciliophora subphylum, the Ciliate class (Ciliata). increase.

Type: Infusoria - Infusoria ciliophora Class: Ciliated infusoria - Ciliata
Category: Homociliates - Holotricha
Representative: Infusoria slipper - Paramecium caudatum

Objective : To consolidate knowledge by studying the structure, nutrition, and movement of the infusoria slipper through experiments.
Equipment needed: Slippery elm culture, slipper plate, microscope, hand magnifying glass, specimen and cover glass, dropper, NaCl, acetic acid
a mixture of methyl green solutions, gelatin solution, filter paper, hygroscopic cotton, and a straightening needle.
Theoretical part: The cnidaria is the most common freshwater cnidaria, with a diameter ranging from 0.2-0.35 mm to 1 mm . The cnidaria is a unicellular organism, consisting of an external ectoplasm and an internal endoplasm.

The upper surface of the pellicle is covered with an extremely large number of identical cilia. covered with. They perform the function of movement. Under the pellicle are hair-like trichocytes that protrude like threads when exposed to various stimuli. They perform a protective function. In the central part of the body of the shoe, there are 2 large (macronucleus) and small (micronucleus) nuclei there is.

the digestive organoids is as follows: in the anterior half of the abdominal side there is a pre- mouth recess (peristome), at the bottom of which there is a hole that connects with the pharynx-cytopharynx . Its other end opens into the endoplasm.

The food that has passed into the endoplasm forms a digestive vacuole . This vacuole gradually separates from the pharynx and begins to move in the endoplasm, and then a new vacuole appears in its place . Digestion

Undigested food residues are removed from the cytoplasm through a special excretory opening of the body - the pore . The shoe has two contractile vacuoles. One is located on the front side, and the second is located on the lower side of the body. Contractile vacuoles perform the function of osmoregulation . The shoe releases fluid equal to the volume of its body through its vacuoles for 40-50 minutes. Contractile vacuoles contract 3 times (in turn) in 1 minute at a temperature of 16 ^{o}. The shoe reproduces in 2 ways , namely sexually and It reproduces in a sexless way .

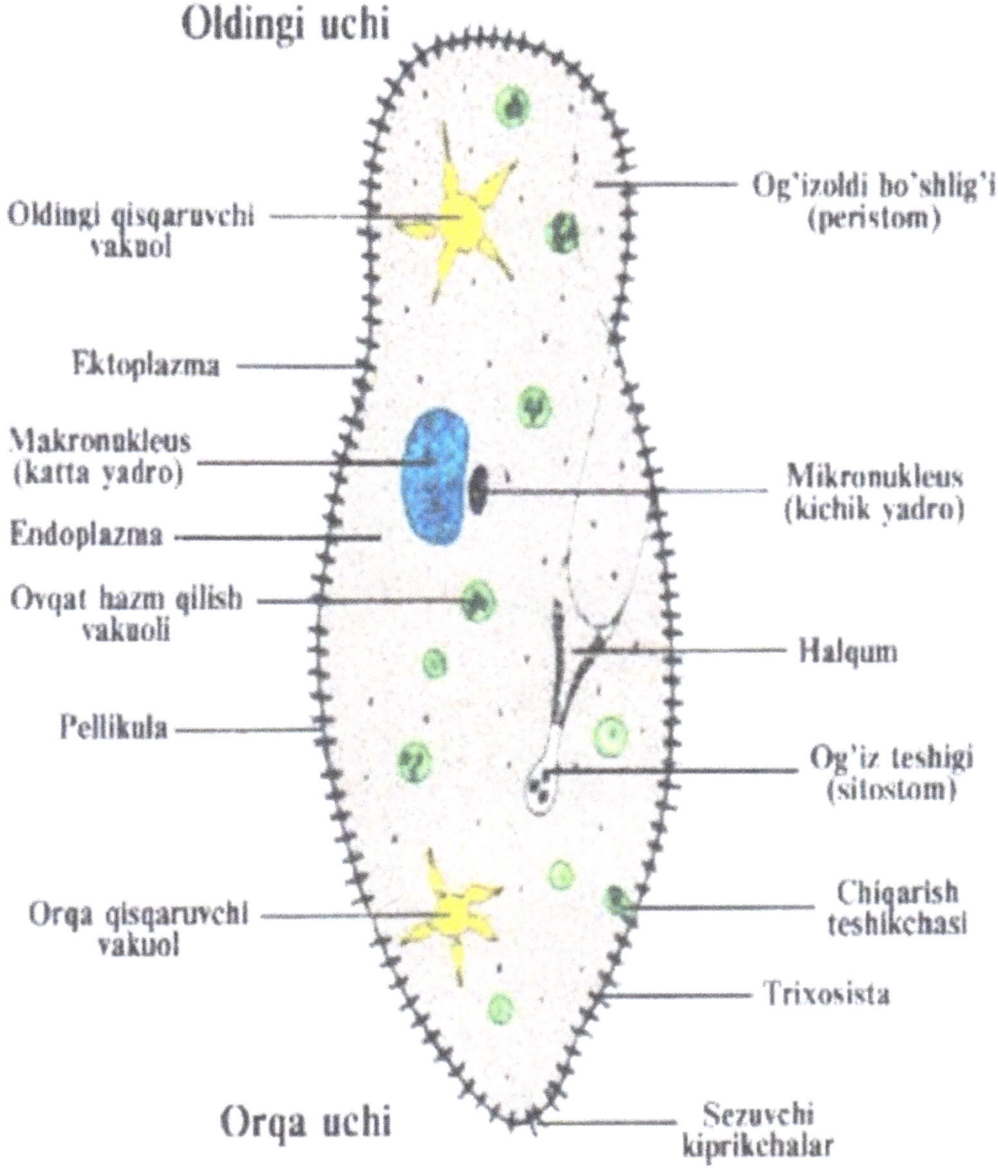

7. Structure of the infusorian slipper

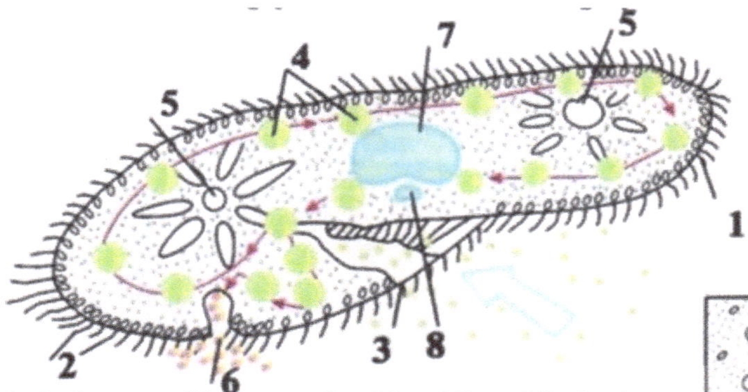

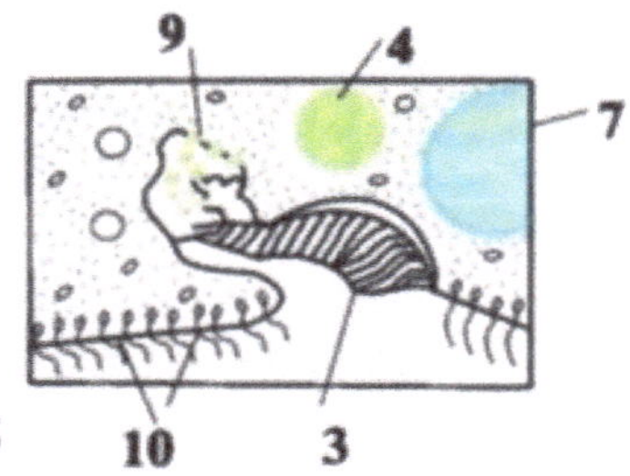

1- hujayra qobig'i
2- kiprikchalari
3- og'izchasi
4- hazm vakuolalari
5- qisqaruvchi vakuola
6- chiqarish teshikchasi
7- katta yadro
8- kichik yadro
9- hazm qilish vakuolasining shakllanishi
10- otiluvchi tanacha

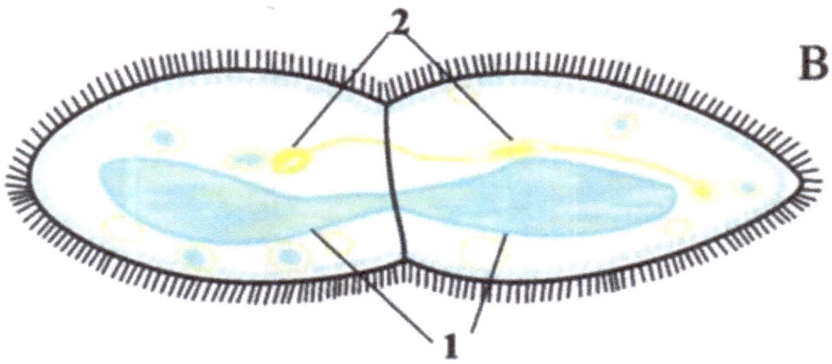

1- bo'linayotgan katta yadro
2- bo'linayotgan kichik yadro

8-. A-shoe structure and nutrition,

Asexual reproduction of B-shoes

Working procedure :

1. **Experiment** . The movement of the slipper observation.

To do this, 1 drop of culture is placed on the slide , a coverslip is placed over it , and the prepared preparation is observed under a small objective. On one side of the body white, formed as a result of the movement of the infusoria, a little It is possible to observe the inward turning . This is a pre-oral turning, called a peristome.

2. **Experiment** . To observe the body structure and digestion of a moving frog, we slow down the movement of a moving frog using one of the following methods:

a) Place several cotton fibers in a row on the slide, add 1 drop of culture and cover the slide. The excess water between the slide and the coverslip is again blotted with paper . The movement of the infusoria caught between the cotton fibers slows down. As a result, observation becomes easier.

b) To remove water from the culture, pieces of filter paper are placed between the object and the cover glass. The water should not be removed completely , otherwise the infusoria may be crushed between the glasses and die. possible.

, 1 drop of the congarot or gelatin solution prepared in a watch glass is dropped onto the specimen glass and, using one of the above methods, its movement is slowed down and its body structure is studied under a large objective. The organoids of the slipper in the congarot solution are well it seems.

The spherical digestive vacuoles are clearly visible in the endoplasm of the shoe. Since the shoe absorbs food (bacteria) along with the pigment , the vacuoles are blue (acidic) or red (alkaline) in color, depending on the environment. will be.

Observing the process of digestion of food in the digestive vacuole , we know that the vacuoles initially have an acidic and then an alkaline environment, because when food passes from the "pharynx" to the vacuole, the vacuole becomes very pale. begins.

3. **Experiment** . The nuclear apparatus and influence of the shoe. observation.

To do this, 1 drop of the culture is placed on the slide, a drop of metallic green mixture is added, and the coverslip is closed.

In this process, the nuclear apparatus appears green . When exposed to acetic acid or NaCl , the infusoria slipper dies, throwing its long, irregular filaments in different directions. These filaments are trichocytes, i.e. protective is an organ.

Assignments on the topic.

1. Using a microscope, draw the outline of the movement of the infusoria in your notebook. 2. Using a microscope, draw the organoids observed in the shoe. to your notebook

Draw.

In your notebook, record the green-stained nucleus of the slipper under the influence of methyl green , and the trichocytes exposed to salt and acid. Draw.

Control questions:

1. What is the structure of the infusorian slipper?

1. Where are the infusoria slippers ? lives?
2. The feeding, movement and reproduction of the slipper Explain?
3. How long does it take for contractile vacuoles to contract? is it worth?
4. The function of contractile vacuoles Explain?
5. Systematic position of the infusoria slipper Tell me?

5- Laboratory exercise.

Subject: Structure, movement, nutrition and reproduction of the Aurelia jellyfish, a representative of the class Scyphozoa .

Phylum: Coelenterata Class: Cyphoid jellyfish -Scyphozoa
Representative: Aurelia aurita - Aurelia aurita

The purpose of the work: to study the nutrition and movement of Aurelia through virtual laboratories and videos, and to consolidate knowledge.

Required equipment : Aurelia fixed in a 5% solution of formalin mixed with seawater , plates showing their structure and reproduction, Petri dishes, tweezers , hand magnifying glasses , preparation needles, Congo violet or red stain, rectangular or circular pieces of black paper cut out , droppers, straightening needle, syringe, water.

Theoretical part: Aurelia is widespread in the Arctic, Barents, White and Far Eastern seas . Its umbrella-shaped body is not very large , up to 20-30 cm in diameter. On the edge of the umbrella are about a hundred large tentacles , and between them are 8 coastal bodies-rhopalia (Fig. 20-21). Among them are small light-sensitive eyes, an organ of balance and olfactory nerve cells

of the umbel there are 4 preoral lobes (palpators), and in the middle of them is a rectangular mouth (Fig. 21). All the palps in front of the mouth and around the umbel have efferent cells. A short pharynx, which continues after the mouth, joins the central part of the gastrovascular system, that is, the stomach . The stomach forms 4 chambers separated from each other by a membrane. These are the gastric filaments, which have a large number of efferent and glandular cells. there is.

Eight branching and eight unbranching radial canals begin from the gastric chambers and join the circular canal at the edge.

The inner surface of all canals is covered with ciliated cells. Due to the movement of these cilia, water and nutrients are constantly moving throughout the gastrovascular system of the aurelia. flowing In this case , food moves from the stomach to the annular canal through unbranched channels, and vice versa through branched channels. Thus, the channels of the gastrovascular system supply the jellyfish's rather large body with food, while oxygen enters along with the water, from which the jellyfish breathes, and waste products are excreted along with the water. goes

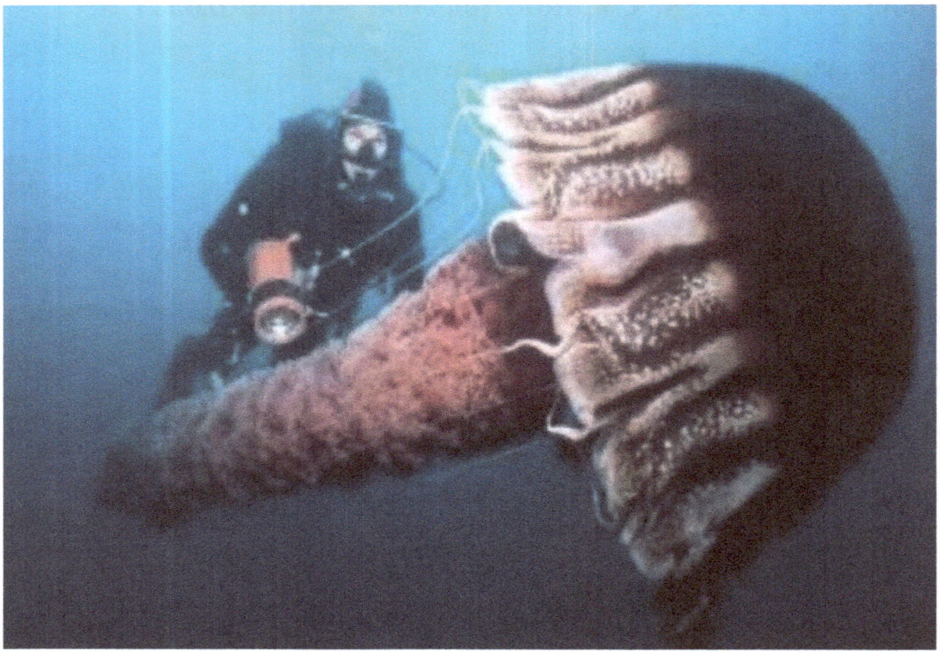

9 . Scyphoid jellyfish structure

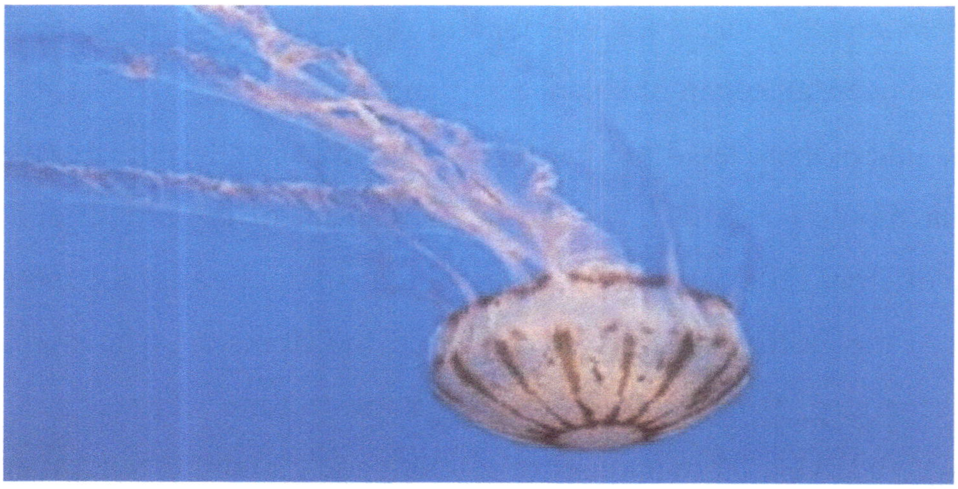

10.Scyphoid structure

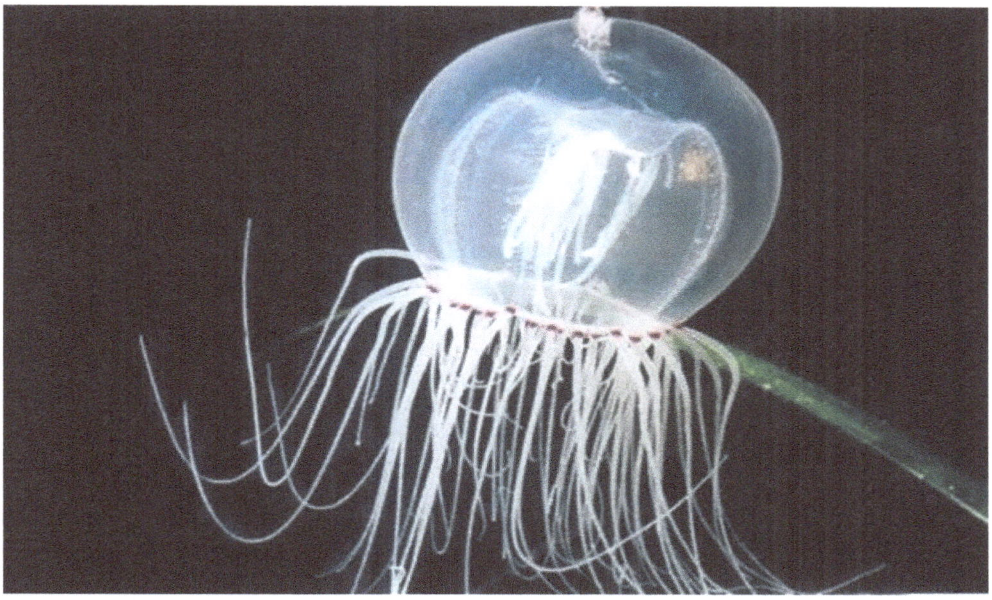

11.Scyphoid jellyfish. A-Ildizogiz jellyfish structure

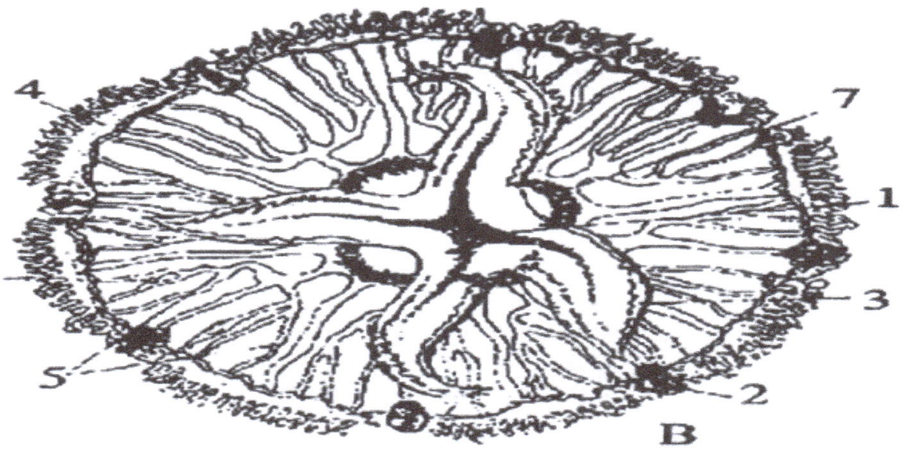

12. Scyphoid

A-Rootmouth jellyfish. B-Aurelia. 1-mouth, 2-rhopalia, 3-mouth segments, 4-annular tube, 5-radial tubes, 6-tentacles, 7-gonads

of Aurelia , mature eggs and sperm pass into the channels of the gastrovascular system , then into the stomach, and from there they are expelled through the mouth (Fig. 28). In some jellyfish , the egg is fertilized in water , but in Aurelia, after the eggs are released from the mouth , they fall into the chambers of the gill slits on its preoral fins and are fertilized there. The fertilized egg breaks down, goes through the blastula and gastrula stages, and turns into a larva - planula , covered with cilia . After the planula floats freely for a long time , it sinks to the bottom of the sea and turns into a sedentary - scyphostoma . It first has 4, then 8, and finally 16 tentacles . will be.

Scyphistoma reproduces by budding and can form new scyphistomas . The transverse division of the scyphistoma produces ring-shaped joints , and the scyphistoma turns into a strobila consisting of several rings . These rings gradually separate from the strobila and, in their structure , form ephyrae, similar to jellyfish , which, in turn, turn into small jellyfish while swimming . Thus, in scyphomedusae , asexual reproduction (scyphistoma) and sexual reproduction (medusae) joints are combined stands.

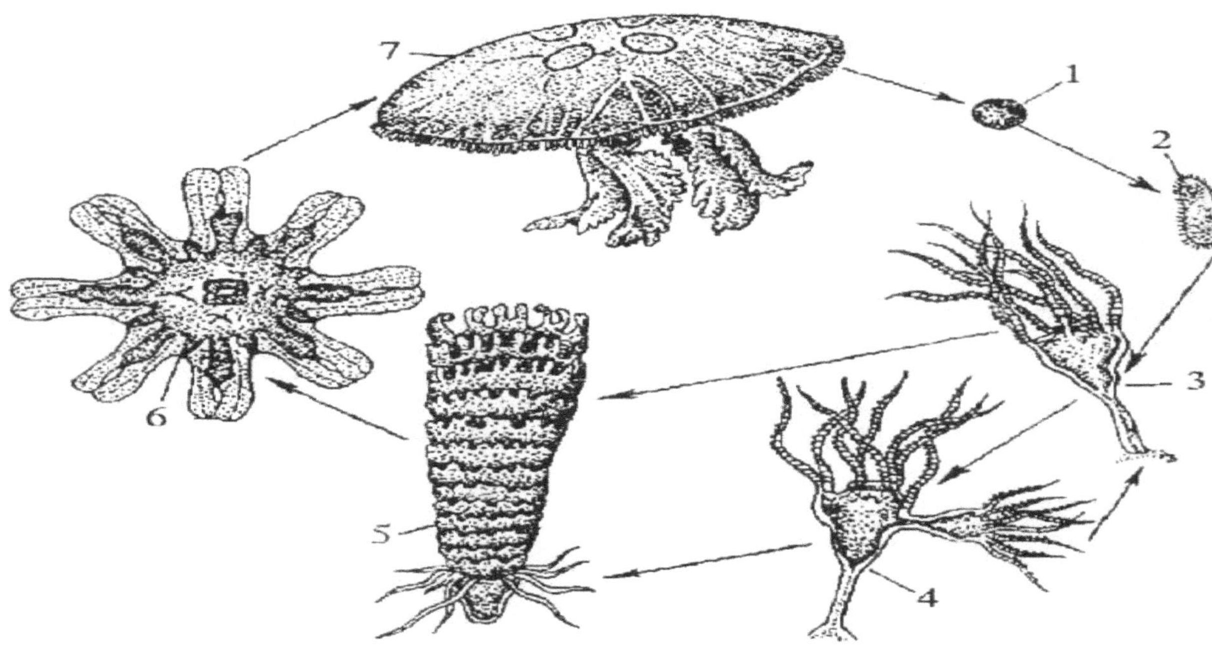

13.Development of xiphoid jellyfish1 - egg, 2 - planula larva, 3 - scyphistompolyp, 4 - budding scyphistome,5 - lateral division of the sifistome, 6 - young spiracle, 7 - mature spiracle.

Work order:

1. To study the structure of Aurelia, small jellyfish are taken, placed in a Petri dish, placed on pieces of black paper , and observed using a hand magnifying glass . Pay attention to the structure of the radial canals and rhopalia give.
2. With the subumbrella of Aurelia's umbrella-shaped body facing up , draw the preoral lobes and mouth opening. find.
3. of the Aurelia umbrella by the handle , slowly stretch it to both sides and with a dropper, inject a diluted solution of purple or red blood dye through the mouth of the jellyfish with extreme caution (otherwise the tubes may burst). Observe the channels of the gastrovascular system according to the spread of the color. Drawing of the structure of Aurelia and the stages of reproduction Draw.

Assignments on the topic .

1. The structure of the jellyfish watch.
2. Draw the appearance of a jellyfish in your notebook. Draw.
3. Aurelia, put a picture of your organs in your album, which you saw in the outline. Download.

Control questions:

1. Structure and size of the Aurelian jellyfish How much?
2. of the Aurelian jellyfish structured? 3. What is the nervous system of the Aurelian jellyfish? structured?
4. the Aurelia jellyfish like? increases?

6- Laboratory exercise.

Topic: External and internal structure of the white planaria (Dendrocoelum lacteum), a representative of the phylum Platyhelminthes, class Turbellaria. increase.

Type: Flatworms - Plathelminthes Class: Ciliated worms - Turbellaria Category: Planarians - Tricladida Representative: White planaria - Dendrocoelum lacteum

Purpose of the work:

consolidate knowledge by studying fixed, stained preparations of white planaria

Equipment needed: Live and fixed planaria, stained planaria preparation, microscope, preparation and hand loupes, watch and specimen glass, needle, dropper, and water.

Theoretical part : White planaria lives in slow-moving, clear waters rich in algae and humus, under rocks in ditches.

The body of the planaria is tubular , 15-26 mm in size . It is covered on the upper side with ciliated epithelium . Due to the cilia moving in a uniform manner in water, the planaria is provided with oxygen . The movement of the planaria occurs with the help of longitudinal and transverse muscles that form the skin-muscle sac , and a mucous fluid produced by unicellular glands in the skin. Therefore, it moves with wave-like movements moves.

The head of the planarian is slightly compressed, and a pair of eyes are located on its shoulder (indicating that it is a bilaterally symmetrical animal).

The digestive system begins at the mouth and ends at the pharynx. The pharynx is three-horned, and its last end is connected to the cecum. There is no anal opening. Undigested food remains are expelled directly through the mouth.

Below the ciliated cells are two layers of circular and longitudinal muscle cells. The ciliated cells and muscle layers form the wall of the skin-muscle sac. Planaria moves by gliding slowly with the help of cilia or by rising to the surface of the water and swimming.

The circular muscles allow movement, while the longitudinal muscles allow bending of the body. In addition, the erector spinae muscles, which extend from the back to the abdomen, help flatten the body.

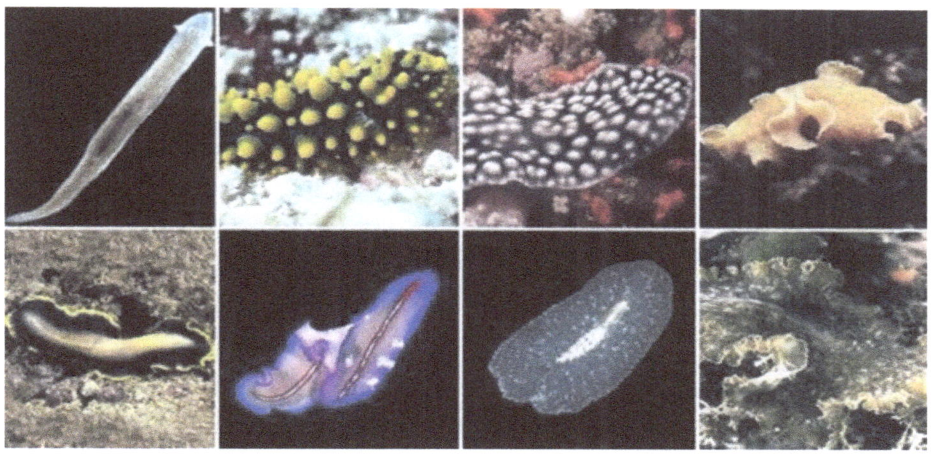

14. Diversity of ciliated worms

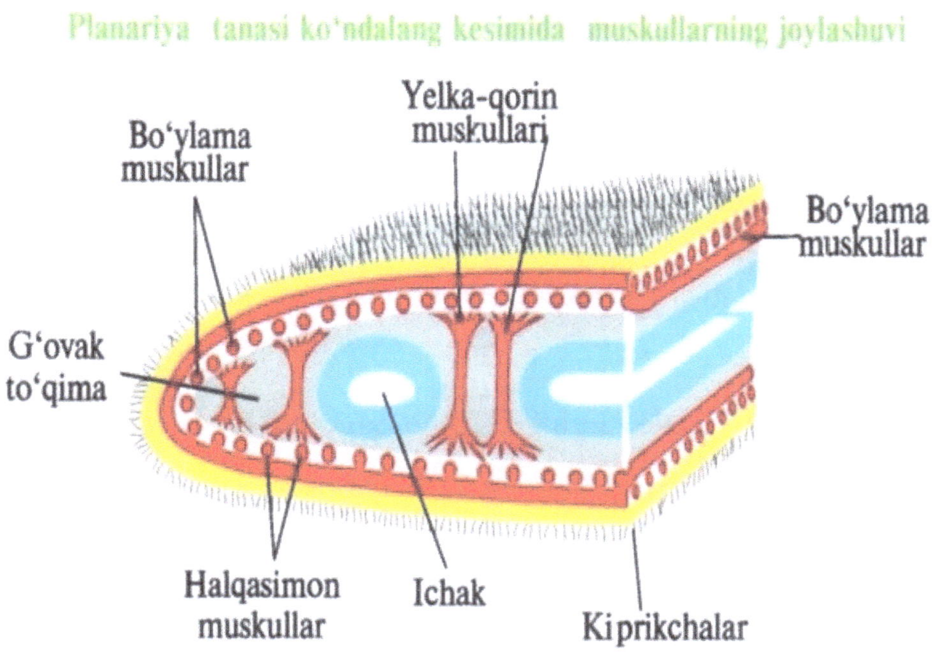

15. Muscle arrangement of the white planaria

The nervous system of the white planaria consists of a nerve ganglion located near the head and a series of nerve fibers running downwards. These nerves are connected to each other by transverse commissures.

Excretory organs consist of protonephridial- like terminal cells. consists of.

Planarians are hermaphroditic, but during reproduction, both sexes join and exchange sperm . Fertilized eggs They are wrapped in cocoons and attached to various objects in the water. puts.

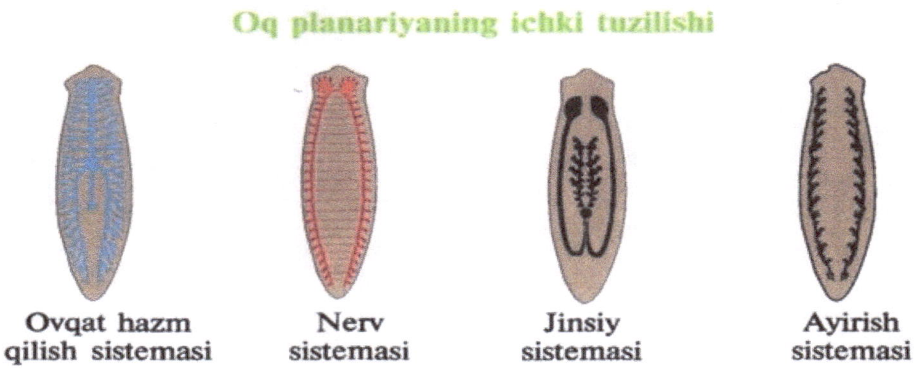

Figure 16. Internal structure of the white planaria.

Work order:

1. in the water in a watch glass and observe its movement using binoculars or a hand-held magnifying glass. Note that when you touch the planaria's body with a needle, it contracts and then slowly returns to its original shape. give.
2. Place a live planaria in a drop of water on a slide and cover it with a coverslip with wax or plasticine legs . Observe the movement of the planaria's cilia first through the small and then through the large objective lenses of the microscope. watch.
3. the dissecting needle slightly on the edge of the coverslip , slow down the movement of the planaria as much as possible and observe the digestive system using binoculars . If live planaria are not available, ready-made stained micropreparations of planaria can also be used for this purpose .
4. General view of the white planaria , a diagram of the schematic structure of the digestive and nervous systems Draw.

Assignments on the topic .

1. the shape of the planarian and draw it in your notebook. Draw.

2. spot on the front of the planarian and draw the outline in your notebook . Move the prepared slide and find the three horns, the mouth, the muscular pharynx , and the genital opening , and draw the outline in your notebook. Draw.

Control questions :

1. Systematic position of white planaria Tell me?
2. Living conditions of planaria and spread?
3. The structure of the planaria how?
4. What is a planarian ? moves?
5. What is a planarian ? increases?
6. digestive system of a planarian Explain?

7- Laboratory exercise.

Topic: External and internal structure of the common liver fluke (Fasciola hepatica), a representative of the Trematoda class, as well as the structure and development processes of the reproductive system of flukes . The structure and development

Phylum: Flatworms – Plathelminthes Class: Flukes – Trematoda

Subclass: Digenetic tapeworms - Digenea Representative: Liver fluke - Fasciola hepatica Work purpose:

Posters and ready-made illustrations depicting the external and internal structure of the liver fluke strengthening knowledge using drugs

Required equipment: Plates depicting the structure of the liver fluke, stained micropreparation of the liver fluke, fixed (in alcohol) liver fluke, steamed glass and hand loupes, microscope, watch and specimen glass, scald glass, tweezers.

Theoretical part: The liver fluke or fasciola is a parasite that infects the liver of various small and large cattle, as well as other herbivorous animals. It can sometimes be found in humans. It lives in the bile ducts of the liver and feeds on blood and products produced in the liver.

The body is bilaterally symmetrical, reaching a length of 2-3 cm. In the middle of the conically elongated anterior sucker is the mouth, and below it on the ventral side is the abdominal sucker. These suckers attach to the bile ducts and serve as a support. The skin-muscular sheath of the suckers is also similar to that of ciliated worms, but the body of trematodes, including the liver fluke, is also covered with a cytoplasmic coat called the tegument. These two , i.e. consists of an outer layer without a core and an inner layer with a core.

The outer and inner layers of the tegument are separated by a plasma membrane. The cytoplasm beneath the membrane contains several small vacuoles, as well as mitochondria and small hairs consisting of cuticle. exists.

The underside of the outer layer of the tegument is covered with a basement membrane, through which tiny pores with ore cytoplasmic threads pass, connecting the two layers of the tegument to each other.

digestive system of the liverworm begins with the mouth, located in the middle of the sucker in the anterior part of the body . After the mouth, the pharyngeal cavity and the pharynx, all of which together form the food- absorbing apparatus . The midgut, which develops from the endoderm, divides into two main branches , which in turn form several lateral blind outgrowths. does.

No anal opening, food waste is excreted through the mouth is released.

The underside of the outer layer of the tegument is covered with a basement membrane , through which tiny pores pass cytoplasmic threads with ore, connecting the two layers of the tegument to each other. stands.

digestive system of the liverworm begins with the mouth, located in the middle of the sucker in the anterior part of the body . After the mouth, the pharynx and the pharynx, all of which together form the food- sucking apparatus . The midgut, which develops from the endoderm, is divided into two main branches , which in turn form several lateral blind outgrowths. There is no anal opening, and food remains are excreted through the mouth. is released.

The excretory organs are arranged in the form of protonephridia . In the middle of the body there is a collecting duct , which is joined by several small collecting ducts . The main excretory duct is located at the posterior end of the body. opens outwards.

The circulatory and respiratory systems are not developed. The nervous system is poorly developed compared to ciliated worms . Three pairs of longitudinal nerve fibers (abdominal, dorsal and lateral) extend from the prepharyngeal nerve ganglion to the oral sucker and the posterior end of the body . These nerve fibers are interconnected by commissures . In most suckers, including liverworms , there is no ootype. In this case, the ootype functions at the end of the ovary, which is the excretory organ release of yolk sacs into the enlarged part

The tube joins . The small unicellular glands covering this part of the ovary from above form the Melis corpuscle. The fertilized eggs are covered with yellow substance here and are attached to the post. is covered.

In this part of the ovary begins a very twisted organ - the uterus. It becomes thinner in front of the abdominal sucker and opens into the genital cloaca. During the mating of the liverworms, spermatozoa pass through the uterus, which also acts as a vagina. In the mature liverworm, the fertilized eggs are stored in the uterus and the initial period of development begins there. spends it on the ground.

, which form numerous small branches and are located in the central part of the body of the liverworm . The seminal ducts from each testis join together near the abdominal sucker, forming a seminal vesicle , which then turns into a thin vas deferens. This opens into the cirrus, the organ of copulation. The cirrus is usually located inside the cirrus sac , which is only turned outward during copulation. comes out.

Development. The liver fluke is a hermaphroditic animal. Its fertilized eggs are released from the bile ducts of the host's liver into the intestines and from there into the external environment with feces. If the eggs fall into water, they hatch into microscopic, ciliated larvae called "miracidia."

The larvae swim for a while in the water . Then, after collecting freshwater mucus , they enter its body , shed their cilia and enter the second larval stage, the redia . The larvae begin to multiply as they develop inside the mucus. These larvae grow and develop into the third larval stage, the cercariae . The cercariae have tails will be.

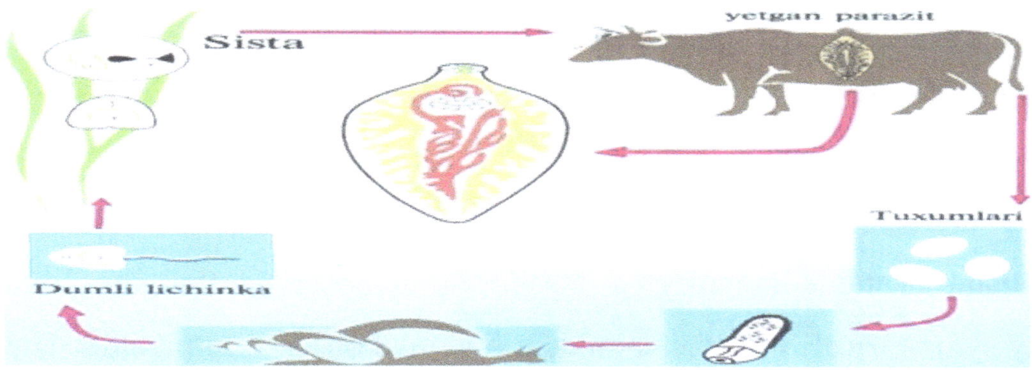

Chuchuk Water Eyelashes

17.Development of liver fluke cyclical

They emerge from the mollusk's body into the water, swim for a while, shed their tail, and become a cyst. The cysts can float on the surface of the water or attach to plants. When these cysts enter the intestines of animals with water or food, the cyst shell dissolves. The larvae hatch in the intestinal cavity. They travel through the intestinal wall through the blood to the liver, attach to the bile ducts, and become parasitic.

Thus , the liver fluke develops in two organisms . When it reaches sexual maturity, it parasitizes in the bile ducts of various livestock and wild animals, and sometimes the liver of humans. Therefore, humans and mammals are the main hosts of the liver fluke. is considered.

The parasite larva lives in the body of a water snail. The water snail is the intermediate host of the liver fluke. The liver fluke is a parasite of livestock and domestic animals.

It is a common and dangerous parasite. A person can also become infected with liver fluke by drinking from puddles in the field or by eating grass in the pasture.

Work order:

1. The fixed liverworm is placed on a watch or glass slide and examined using a hand or table magnifying glass . It is observed that the liverworm is bilaterally symmetrical, with the shoulders flattened on the ventral side. The oral and abdominal suckers and the genital opening between them are visible. to find.

2. view the internal organs, a specially stained preparation is used, showing the digestive , excretory, and reproductive systems . The prepared micropreparation is examined under a magnifying glass . is observed.

Assignments on the topic .

1. Observe the external structure of the liver fluke. Add the picture to the album. Draw.
2. the internal structure of the liver fluke in your notebook and draw a picture of it.

Control questions: 1. Systematic position of the liver fluke? 2. Structure of the liver fluke how?

3. the liver fluke parasitize? 4. Explain the reproduction of the liver fluke? 5. Describe the nutrition of the liver fluke Explain?

8-Laboratory training

Topic: Representatives of the class of tapeworms (Cestoda) - cattle tapeworm (Taeniarhynchus saginatus) and pig The structure and development of tapeworms (Taenia solium). The structure and development of some representatives of tapeworms development

Type: Flatworms – Plathelminthes Class: Tapeworms - Cestoidea
Representative: Cattle tapeworm (cattle tapeworm) - Taeniarhynchus sagianatus .

Purpose of the work:

Reinforce knowledge using posters and prepared preparations and wet preparations depicting the external and internal structure of the bovine tapeworm

Equipment needed : Cattle tapeworm, plate depicting scolex , plates depicting mature and hermaphrodite proglattides, wet preparation of cattle tapeworm, head, microscopic preparation of mature hermaphrodite segments, microscope, dissecting knife, and hand loupes, bandage, tweezers, petri dish.

Theoretical part : Tapeworms are almost parasitic forms . The sexually mature forms are parasitic inside vertebrates. They do not have a digestive organ. The body consists of a head-scolex, neck and strobiles (Figure 35).

The cattle tapeworm lives in the small intestine of humans. This parasite lives in the digested food and feeds by absorbing nutrients with the surface of its body. The tapeworm does not need to be free to reach its adult form, which is why the tapeworm has developed the property of anaerobic dissimilation . Therefore , glycogen in the body parenchyma of the tapeworm plays an important role in their life. The body of the worm is ribbon-shaped, flattened by a white shoulder-abdomen . The length of the tapeworm (T. saginatus) can be up to 10 m, sometimes longer .

The worm has a head, neck and body. The head is spherical, the anterior end is slightly enlarged, and is 1.5-2 mm long. diameter . The scolex has 4 round suckers , located symmetrically on all four sides . The edges of the suckers are thick, because they are rich in muscle . The neck is the growth point (zone). As a result of the transverse division (budding) of the neck, clearly distinguishable joints - proglottids - storbillae are formed one after another . Due to this budding, the body grows. The number of such proglottids in the roundworm can be more than 10 thousand . Proglottids are not the same. The farther the proglottids move from the scolex , the larger they become. The side of the mature joints is shorter than the height. For example, it is 5-7 mm wide and 16-30 mm long . The skin-muscular layer of the worm consists of multilayer cuticle epithelium (covering tissue) and layers of circular and longitudinal muscles . The parenchyma under the skin-muscle sac contains internal organs, the body cavity no.

Life stages of the cattle tapeworm (Taenia)

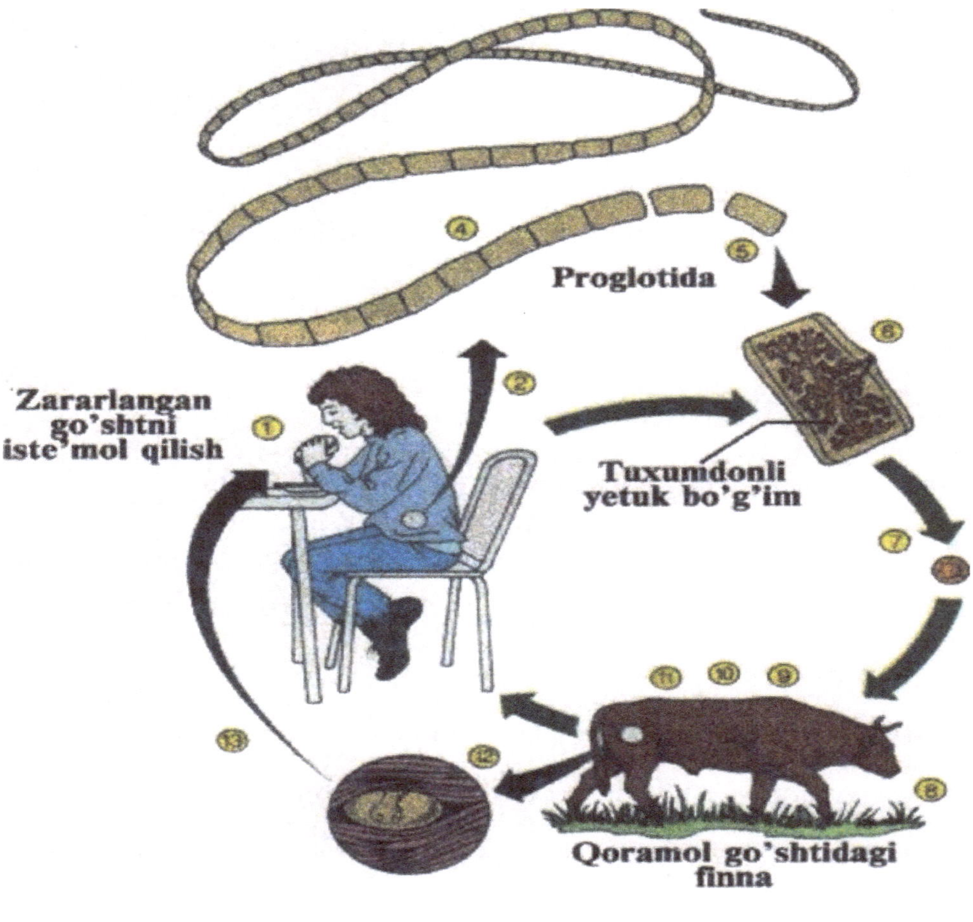

18. Life stages of the cattle tapeworm

No digestive system. It absorbs food with the entire surface of its body. The excretory system consists of nephridial tubes . consists of.

two on each side and lead to the excretory orifice through the excretory bladder. opens.

In the tapeworm, the nervous system consists of a large head node, from which ten nerve "nets" spread out to the joints. The largest of these nerve "nets" are located on either side. Two nerve "nets" cross all the joints along their length. will pass.

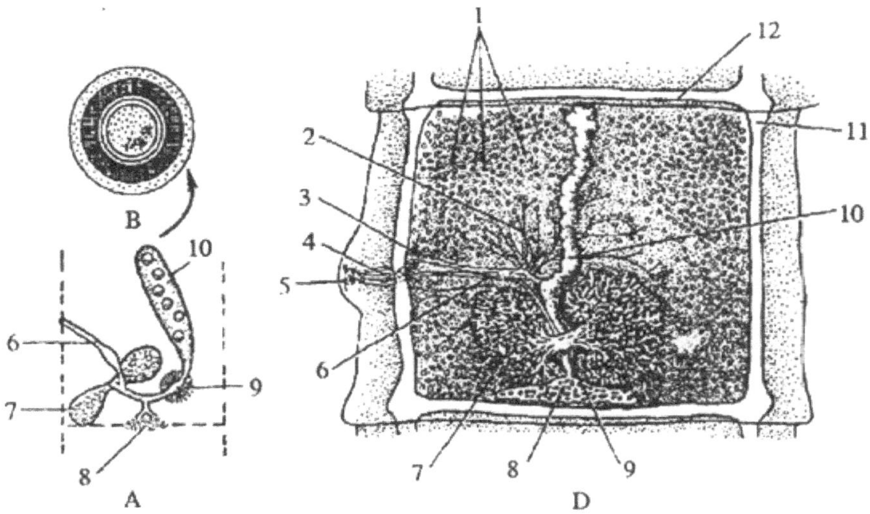

19: The development cycle of the cattle tapeworm.

A - diagram of the structure of the female reproductive system. B - oncosphere egg, D - hermaphrodite joint of the black tapeworm.

Olfactory nerves are mainly located in the suckers . Tapeworms are hermaphrodites. Young joints do not have sexual organs . In joints in 1/3 of the body, it is possible to observe segments with mature sexual organs . This is the case in several sections repeated.

male reproductive organ is the testicles, the copulatory organ, and the genital tract . The testicles are in the form of small vesicles that are scattered throughout the penis . The vas deferens begin from the testicles, which join together to form the vas deferens. does.

The oviduct opens into the external genital opening on the side of the proglottid. The oviduct forms many folds and becomes the oviduct . The oviduct connects to the cereus in the serous sac. The female reproductive gland consists of two ovaries, a yolk sac with scattered oviducts, and the uterus that later forms. enters.

At the very end of the joint, a triangular-shaped yolk sac is connected to the oviduct by the upward-directed yolk sac. At the top of the yolk sac are paired ovules, each ovule connected by a narrow duct and connected to the odd oviduct. The junction of the oviduct and the yolk sac is called the ovule . In this ovule egg they will reach from it

When filled with fertilized eggs, the uterine segment is called a mature segment.

Work order.

1. wet preparation of a tapeworm in a cylindrical container using a hand loupe, paying attention to the shape and size of the proglottids in the anterior, middle, and posterior parts of its body. give.
2. the scolex of the bovine tapeworm stained with carmine through a small microscope objective and note the location of the suckers and the absence of loops . To compare the head of the bovine tapeworm with the structure of the scolex of other solitaires, observe the head of the pig tapeworm and echinococcus under a microscope . Draw a picture of the structure of the scolex of the bovine tapeworm Draw.
3. Observe the microslides of the hermaphrodite segment of the tapeworm, stained with carmine, using binoculars and a small microscope objective . Identify the anterior and posterior sides of the proglottid, where the two-lobed ovary is located. Note the location of the other sexual organs in it . Draw a picture of the hermaphrodite segment Draw.
4. Observe a microscopy of a mature proglottid stained with carmine and note that it is much longer in length than in width . Then, by observing it through a small objective of a binocular or microscope, locate the uterus and its lateral branches . Also note that in such joints most parts of the reproductive system are reduced and draw a picture of it. draw

Assignments on the topic.

1. each proglottid of a tapeworm to each other . Record the width and length in your notebook. take it.

2. Look at the scolex of a tapeworm and draw a picture of it. 3. Distinguish the scolex of the cattle tapeworm from the scolex of other representatives of tapeworms , draw a picture of it. 4. Study the structure of the genital organ and excretory system of a tapeworm and draw a picture of it in your album Draw.

SECOND SEMESTER LABORATORY WORK

Laboratory training.

Subject : Ring phylum Annelida , The structure of the head , tail, and parapodia of Nereis, a member of the class Polychaeta . The sandworm structure

Phylum: Annelids – Annelids Class: Polychaeta – Polychaeta

Representative: Nereis - Nereis

The purpose of the work : To study the topic based on posters and wet preparations depicting the structure, nutrition and development cycle of Nereis , and to stimulate students' cognitive activity. activation.

Required equipment : Nereis structure chart, parapodium chart, Nereis hand-held apparatus, parapodium micro apparatus, microscope, magnifying glass, tweezers, needle, specimen glass, petri dish.

Theoretical part : Nereis is found in the Black, Azov, White and Barents Seas. They live at the bottom of the water , and sometimes in the coastal zone among aquatic plants. Nereis is 10-15 cm long and consists of 80-100 segments . The body is divided into head, trunk and tail (pygidium) . The head consists of two segments , the first segment or prostomium, has 2 pairs of olfactory pits on the lower part, and a pair of tentacles and palps on the anterior side . These are sensory organs. The second segment of the head, the peristomium, is longer and thicker than the other segments . It does not have parapodia , but there are 4 whiskers (cirri) on each side, and the mouth is located on the ventral side. The tail does not have parapodia, but the last segment of the body and the anal opening has a pair of anal tentacles will be.

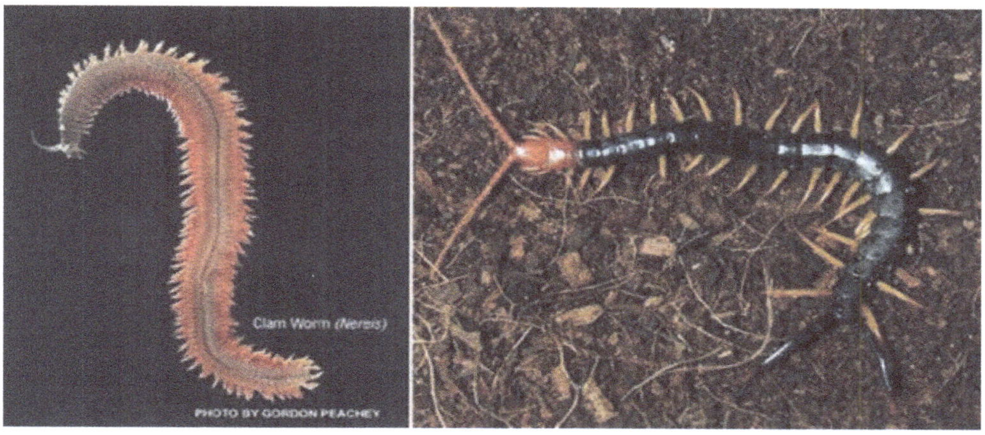

20- Fig. Nereis's exterior structure

the digestive system of the Nereis , that is, the pharynx , is inverted and protrudes outward . Its pair of chitinous jaws, located on its front side and with small holes , capture decaying organic matter and small organisms . Except for the two segments that make up the head of the Nereis, there is a pair of parapodia on the sides of all segments . These are the organs of movement . The parapodia consist of two segments , the shoulder segment of which is called the natopodi, The abdominal segments are called neuropodia. Each of these segments has a single long seta and tufts of hairs (hence the name polychaete worms). Among the hairs on each segment is one very thick hair that protrudes from the base of the parapodia , called the supporting hair - acillus. is called.

Parapodia serve as support when the worm moves underwater, and as paddles when it swims in water.

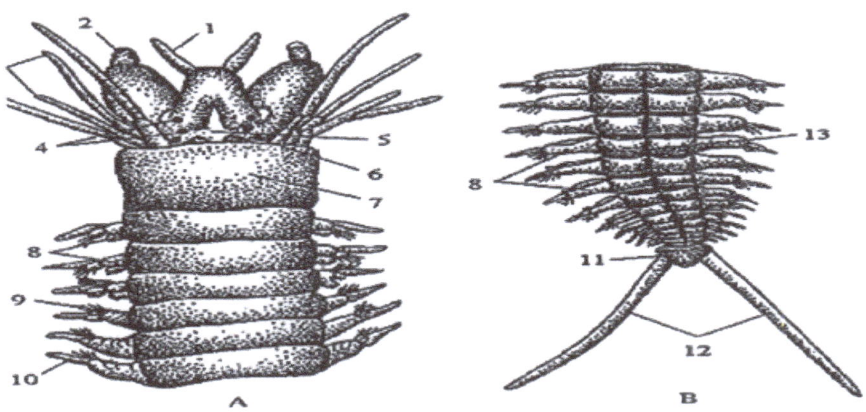

21- Fig. Structure of the head of Nereis . Anterior (A) and posterior (B) of Nereis side.

1 - antennae, 2 - **palp,** 3 - **oral** whiskers, 4 - **skin ,** *5* - **prostomium,** 6 - **olfactory fossa,** 7 - **peristome,** 8 - **parapodia.** 9 - 10 - **posterior whiskers,** 11 - **pygidium,** 12 - **anal whiskers,** 13 - **posterior blood root.**

Procedure . 1. Place 1-2 nereis fixed in formalin solution in a Petri dish and examine their external structure using a hand magnifying glass . Pay attention to the fact that their body consists of the same joints and the parapodia located on their sides . give.

Observe it through a lens, pay attention to the hairs and acicles on its segments, and draw a picture of the structure of the parapodia.

2. the formalin-fixed sandworm in a Petri dish and observe it using a hand magnifying glass. Note its small, basal segments. Note the thinned tail and the absence of parapodia . Describe the general appearance of the tailworm. Draw.

Assignments on the topic .

1. Draw the general appearance of Nereis 2. Draw a picture of Prastomeum

3. Draw a picture of the parapodia of Nereis in your notebook.

Control questions:

1. The systematic position of Nereus Tell me?
2. Where is Nereus? lives?
3. The structure of Nereus Tell me?

10- Laboratory exercise.

Topic : External and internal structure of the earthworm, a representative of the Oligochaeta class structure, skin-muscular sac, movement and reflex. External and internal structure of the medical leech - a representative of the class of leeches (Hirudinea).

Class:Oligochaeta

Representative: Earthworm - Lumbricus rubellus

Purpose of the work: Posters depicting the structure, nutrition and development cycle of an earthworm, to stimulate students' cognitive activity based on the study of living earthworms activation.

Equipment needed : Earthworm reflecting plate, live earthworm , microscope, hand magnifier, cross-section of earthworm, sharp scissors , scalpel, tweezers, needle, bath, water, cotton , and entomological needles.

Theoretical part: The earthworm is 15-20 cm long and lives in soils rich in organic waste. Its body consists of segments with the same structure. The anterior and posterior ends are slightly thinner. The shoulder side is dark, and the abdominal side is whitish. The 32nd-37th segments of its body are much thicker at the shoulder , forming originated from multi-ciliated annelids . As a result of adaptation to living conditions, the parapodia disappeared, and only a part of the cilia remained. remaining.

The segments of the earthworm's body are separated from each other externally by intersegmental ridges, which have holes in them on the worm's shoulders through which body fluid escapes and moistens the skin . This makes it easier for the worm to breathe through its skin .

the earthworm's skin is covered with a very thin cuticle. The epithelium beneath it is covered with circular and longitudinal muscles. All of this forms the worm's skin-muscle sac . The secondary body cavity (coelom), which is characteristic of annelids, is separated from each other on the inside by membranes - dissepiments, corresponding to the body segments . In addition, the cavity in each segment is also divided into right and left parts by the mesentery membrane located under the intestine . The body of the worm is covered with cuticle covered.

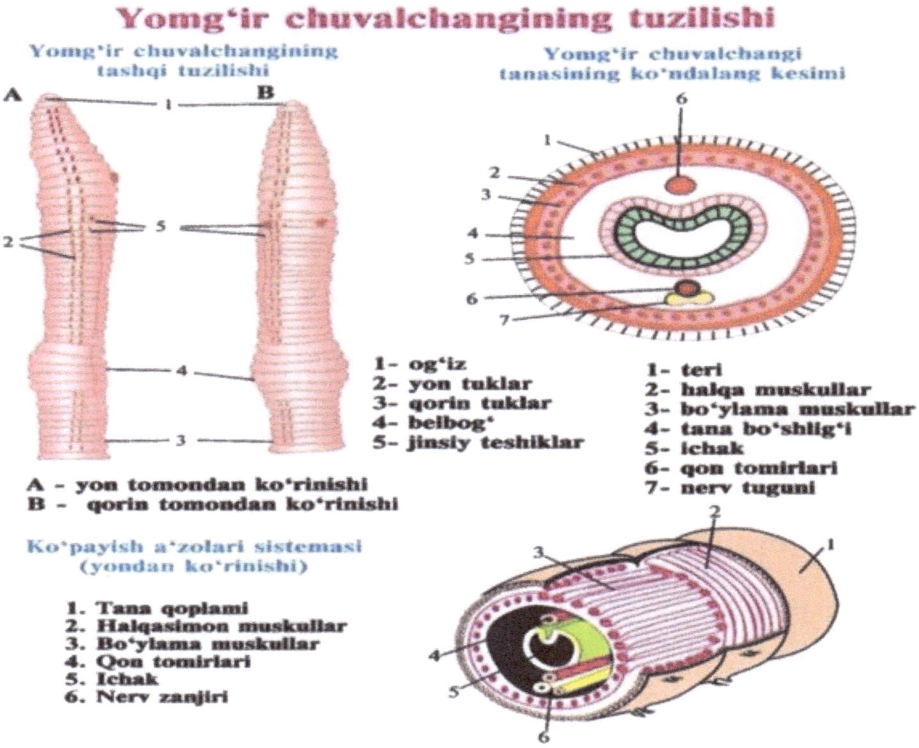

22- **Picture of an earthworm structure** .

Underneath it is the skin, which consists of cylindrical covering tissue (epithelium) cells derived from the endoderm. The skin contains many single-celled glands that produce mucus to keep the skin moist. From the epithelium

then the ring-shaped muscles form a thin layer. The longitudinal muscles are also well developed , forming ribbon-shaped muscles consisting of 4-5 segments. The cuticle, skin and muscle layers together form the cutaneous-muscular sac of the worm . It is separated from the secondary body cavity - the coelom by its wall, the coelothelium or endothelium . Some cells in the skin epithelium form hairs does.

The bristles are made of a substance similar to chitin. They are supported by muscle fibers. Therefore, the bristles can move inward, outward, forward, and backward.

In the middle of the section, a section of the intestine is visible, the upper side of which is covered with coelothelium, which forms the wall of the coelom.

Yomg‘ir chuvalchangining ichki tuzilishi

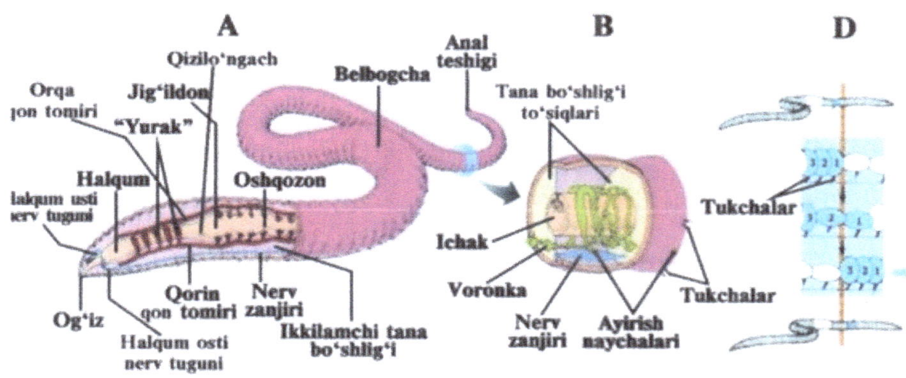

A. Yomg‘ir chuvalchangi tanasi oldingi qismining kesimi
B. Yomg‘ir chuvalchangi tana bo‘g‘imining ichki tuzilishi
D. Yomg‘ir chuvalchangining harakatlanish sxemasi

23- Fig. The interior of an earthworm structure.

In its chloragogenous cells, various excretory substances accumulate in the form of granules . Then these cells break off from the intestinal wall, fall into the coelomic fluid and dissolve. The wall of the midgut is sunken, forming a fold from the back into the intestinal cavity , which is a cephalocele that expands the surface of the intestine for food absorption. Above and below the intestinal section, the sections of the dorsal and

The inner surface of the metonephridial tubes is covered with ciliated epithelial cells. They help to expel waste products. Depending on which part of the worm the section passes through, the nervous system may have different appearances, but the abdominal nerve chain is clearly visible.

Procedure . 1. Clean the live earthworm from mud, place it on a sheet of white paper and distinguish its head, tail, **abdomen** and shoulders from each other. Pay attention to the contraction of the body . If a needle is inserted into the body of the worm, it will move in different directions. Such twisting movements indicate that they have circular and longitudinal muscles . Listen to the sound that the hairs on the segments make when they rub against the paper as the worm moves . You can also feel the presence of hairs by holding the tail of the worm with the thumb and index fingers of your left hand and moving the thumb and index fingers of your right hand from its tail to its head. possible.

2. Using a hand magnifying glass , we can see that the earthworm's body is made up of identical segments and that there are 32-34 segments . located belt part watch.

3. To observe the internal structure of the worm, its movement is first stopped. For this, the worm is immersed in a 15-20% alcohol solution for 15-20 minutes. Then the worm is placed in a bath with the shoulder side facing up and secured by the head and tail with a clamp. Then, a transverse incision is made from the last side of the body using scissors and the skin-muscle sac is cut from the transverse incision towards the head . When opening the skin-muscle sac, the scissors should be held in such a way that the tip of the scissors does not damage the internal organs . Then, holding the body wall with tweezers, the dissepiment membranes are cut using a scalpel and the body wall is fixed to the bath with the clamps . Water is poured until the body of the worm is immersed. After that , observe the internal structure, for this purpose using a hand magnifying glass use.

Case 2 Topic: Structure and development of the medical leech.

Phylum:Annelides - Annelids Subphylum:Clitellata - Clitellata Class: Leeches - Hirudinea Representative: Medicinal leech - Hirudo medicinalis

Purpose of the work: Structure, nutrition and development of the medical leech posters depicting the life cycle , students' knowledge based on studying a living medical leech activate activities.

Required equipment : Tables depicting the morphology, anatomy , and cross-sectional structure of the medical leech, microscopes, hand loupes, sharp-pointed scissors, baths, forceps, containers filled with water , 10° alcohol solution, micropreparations of cross-sectional sections of the leech body in the water live leeches being kept.

Theoretical part:

The medical leech is 15-20 cm long and lives in freshwater bodies. It is an ectoparasite, occasionally sucking blood from aquatic vertebrates or mammals that come close to water, and from humans. Young leeches that have just hatched from eggs also suck blood from fish, aquatic and terrestrial animals.

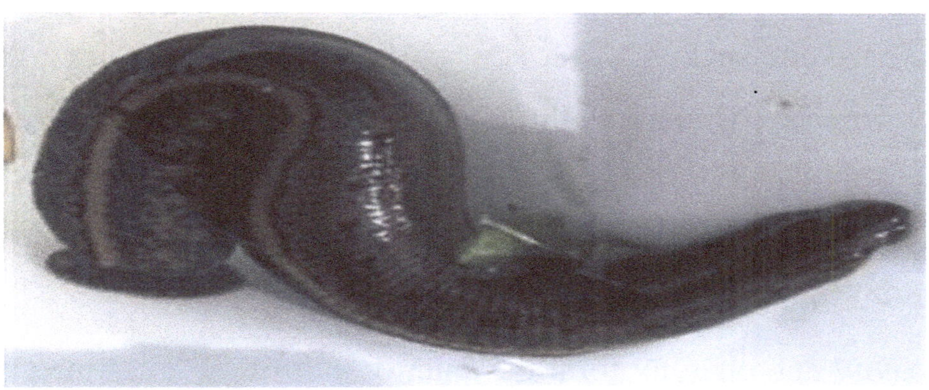

24- Fig. Medicinal leech (Hirudo medicinalis) structure

The body is slightly flattened from the shoulder to the abdominal side. At the anterior end there is a mouth sucker (with a mouth opening in the middle of the sucker), and at the tail there is a much larger anal sucker. The anal opening is located above this sucker. The body of the leech is divided into segments, but these are not true segments, since the number of external joints (102) is not equal to the number of internal joints (33). There are no tentacles or parapodia on the segments, even on the head . There are five pairs of eyes on the shoulder side of the head. The suckers of leeches also serve as an organ of adhesion. The upper part of the skin of leeches is covered with a thin cuticle , under which there are many glands that secrete a mucous substance in a single-layer epithelium. The space between the internal organs is a cavity binder tissue - filled with parenchyma . Leeches do not have a true body cavity, but a secondary cavity - the clavicular system - as a remnant of the coelom exists.

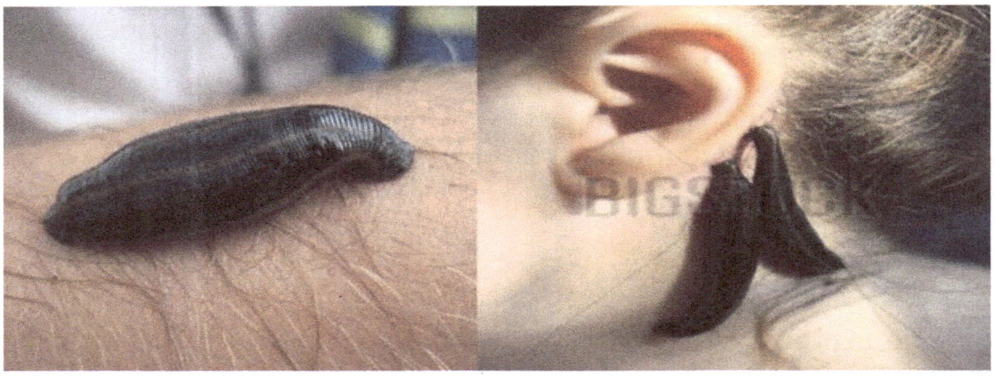

Fig. Medicinal leech (Hirudo medicinalis) structure

The medical leech belongs to the group of jawed leeches; it has 3 jaws made of chitin, located opposite each other , in its oral cavity . Their upper part is jagged, sharpened , and contains 80-90 teeth (Fig. 37). With these, the leeches cut the skin of their host during blood sucking. That is why 3- sided scars remain on the skin after the leech sucks blood . Around the throat of the leech are glands that secrete hirudin fluid. Hirudin fluid prevents blood from clotting, as a result of which it flows continuously while the leech is sucking blood, and blood can flow even after the leech is full .

The oral cavity and pharynx form the anterior part of the intestine , formed from the ectoderm. After it, the midgut or "jellyfish" begins, formed from the endoderm. On both sides of it there are 10-11 pairs of posterior closed outgrowths - diverticula . The last of these outgrowths is long, and it extends to the last end of the body. In these outgrowths, blood mixed with hirudin is stored for a long time without clotting . That is why the leech can live for 11.5 years without sucking blood possible.

The nervous system of the leech consists of supralaryngeal and sublaryngeal nerve ganglia connected to it by connectives , as well as the abdominal nerve chain .

The excretory organs consist of 17 pairs of metanephridia . The medical leech does not have a true circulatory system. Its function is performed by the lacunae system, which is a remnant of the coelom. This system mainly consists of 4 longitudinal canals , which are located on the shoulders, abdomen and both sides. located.

Work order:

1. To examine the external structure of a live or killed leech, use a hand magnifying glass to locate and pay attention to the oral and anal suckers , the colored stripes above

It is fastened and opened by the tail, like an earthworm. opens.

with its digestive system ; carefully observe the pharynx, stomach and hindgut using a hand magnifying glass , paying attention to the segmentation , Remove the digestive system slowly using tweezers . Find the nervous system. Find and count the excretory and reproductive systems. Examine the cross-section of the leech using a small microscope lens; find the skin-muscle sac, the intestine and its side pockets, the lacunae in the circulatory system, and Learn.

Assignments on the topic .

1. General view of the earthworm Draw.
2. Draw in your notebook the location and structure of the spiny legs in different segments.
3. Observe the external structure of a medical leech and draw a picture of it in your album. 4. Observe the internal structure of a medical leech (digestive, nervous, circulatory, gastrointestinal and reproductive organs) and draw a picture of it in your album. Draw.

Control questions:

1. Systematic position of the earthworm Tell me?
2. External structure of an earthworm ?
3. the nervous system of the earthworm structured? 4. The external structure of the medical leech and size?

11- Laboratory exercise.

Topic: Mollusca phylum, Gastropoda class - External and internal structure, movement of freshwater snails or naked snails .

Type: Mollusks - Mollusca

Class: Gastropoda Representative: Helix pomatia

Purpose of the work: To teach students to work and think independently through conducting experiments.

Required equipment : A tapeworm plate, a fixed tapeworm, glass slides, scissors, a straightening needle, a hammer.

Theoretical part: Mollusks are the oldest group of animals with a diverse structure. The upper part of the snail is covered with a shell. Its shell is turned to the right or left. The body is divided into head, legs and caudal parts. The head has a mouth opening and a pair of eyes, and the genital opening opens below the right side of the antenna.

The digestive system of the tapeworm is made up of the foregut, midgut, and hindgut. The respiratory system is made up of the pulmonary lobules.

The circulatory system begins with the heart ventricle, atrium, and atria.

The excretory system consists of a single kidney. The excretory system opens near the respiratory opening. The vine worm is hermaphroditic. It has a single hermaphrodite gland that functions as both an ovary and a testicle . will do.

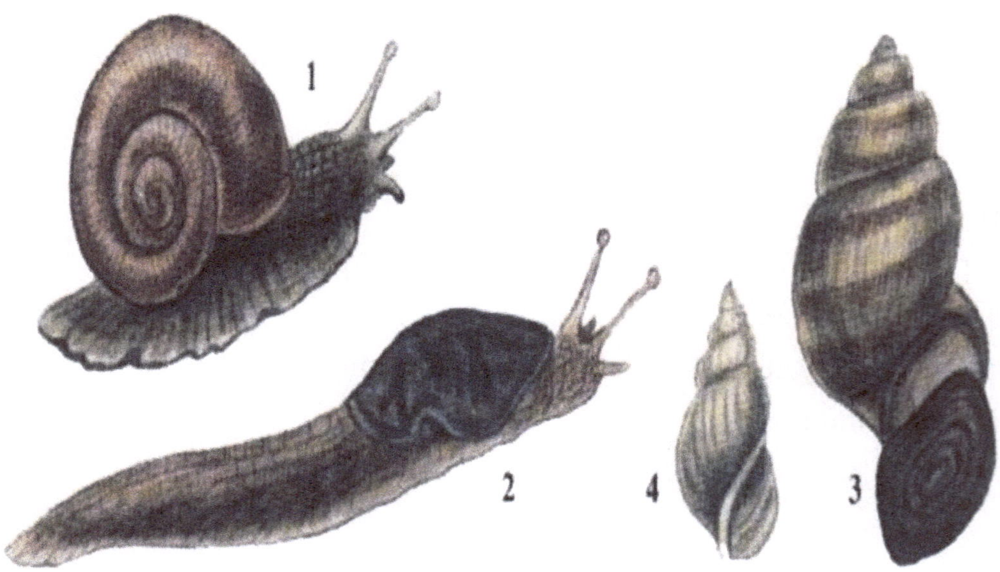

26- picture . Gastropod mollusks :

1 - vine mucus; 2 - naked mucus; 3 - bithynia; 4 - live-bearing mucus.

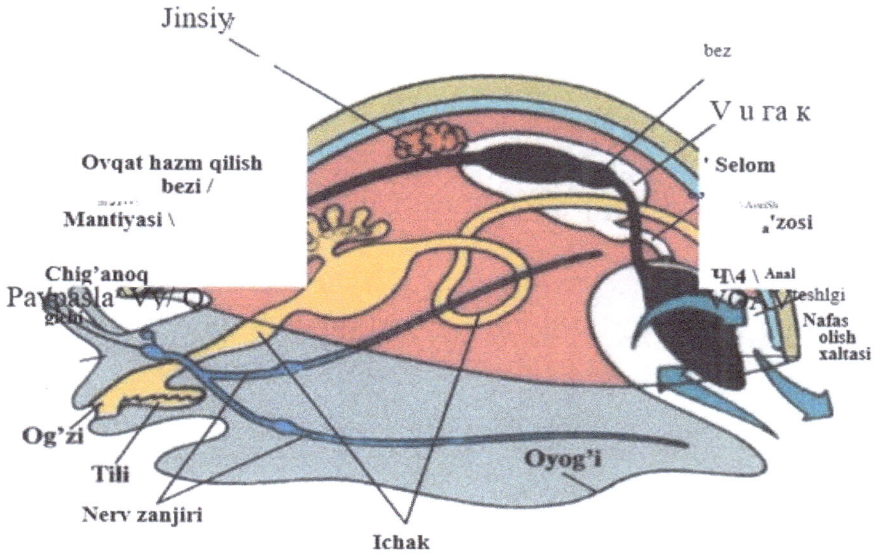

Fig. The inside of a vine slime mold structure

Work order:

1. From a shell separated from the shell to observe its structure and shape is used.
2. Which way is the shell in your hand twisted? define.
3. To observe its movement, a field slime worm is poured into a glass slide and the foot side is placed in a tub from the bottom of the glass slide and the head side is secured with a clamp. The mantle under the shell from the shoulder side is twisted in a spiral like a shell . To open the body, it is cut off from the lung opening by rotating the body above the mantle cavity with scissors . Scissors with heart took bag cut off, heart cameras structure is observed.
4. To view other internal organs, the bottom of the mantle cavity is opened. In this, the body is cut from the last side towards the head, up to the mantle cavity and the head is also cut in two . This cut is cut parallel to the other side , and the cut formed in the middle is removed with tweezers . The larynx, which starts from the mouth, is the esophagus and the head ganglion lying on it, the subpharyngeal ganglion, the salivary gland duct is observed.

Assignments on the topic.

1. The structure and shape of the shell of the vine slime worm draw

2. the slime mold in your notebook , the direction of the wave left by its muscular legs on a clear glass. Draw.

Control questions:

1. What is the external structure of the tapeworm? 2. What is the systematic position of the tapeworm?

3. What is the feeding and respiratory system of the tapeworm ? structured?

12. Laboratory Exercise.

Topic: The main features of the external and internal structure of the clam, a representative of the class of bivalve mollusks (Bivalvia).

Type: Soft-bodied animals Mollusca Class: Bivalve mollusks - Bivalvia

Representative: Toothless mollusk - Anadonta sygnea

Purpose of the work: To teach students to work and think independently through conducting experiments.

Required equipment: live anaconda, warm (45-50 ^{0}) water, gloves, bathtubs, anaconda shells, forceps, scalpels, scissors, entomological forceps, preparation needles, plates depicting the external and internal structures of anaconda, wet preparation of a split anaconda.

Theoretical part: Anadonta lives at the bottom of freshwater reservoirs, rivers and lakes , with the front of its body buried in sand or mud . In the same waters , a similar adapada is also found, but its shell is longer, and the shells are connected to each other by a groove and a tooth called a "lock" . The shell of the Anadon is such devices

It wouldn't be, that's why they call it "toothless".

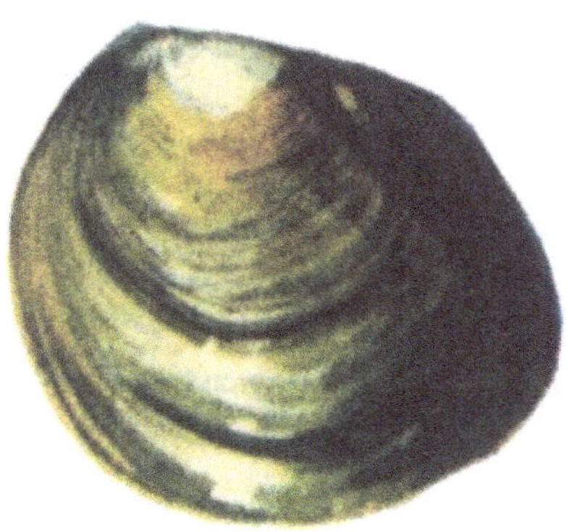

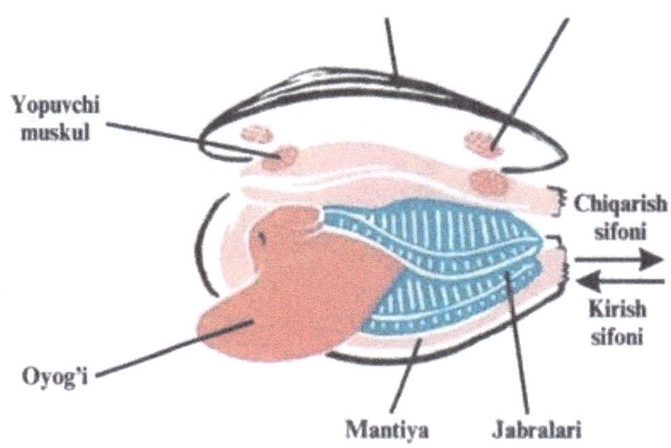

A) Chit exactly B) Closing

28- Fig. External and internal structure of the bivalve The place of attachment of the muscle is located between the body of Anadonta bivalve . This periods

The shoulder is connected by elastic ligaments - ligaments, two, anterior and posterior closing muscles - retractors . The lower side of the shell is open , and a muscular "foot" protrudes from it . With the help of the foot, the anadont moves very slowly on the bottom of the water. The shell , like the front of the shell, is wider, and the back end is thinner. The shell of the anadont, like other mollusks, is made of three layers consists of.

The top layer is made of a horn-like substance called conchialine , in which annual rings can be seen. The other two layers, the calcareous and nacreous parts, are made of limestone .

membrane, which covers the inner surface of the shell, surrounds the body of the anodonta from above and on the sides. A mantle cavity is formed between the mantle membrane and the body . This cavity is open in the anterior part of the body, on the ventral side and at the posterior end , and is called the shell, and when the shells are closed, the edges of the mantle membrane are also tightly closed. it comes together.

As a result, the mantle cavity is separated from the external environment. The mantle membrane is an organ specific to mollusks , which performs functions such as forming the shell and ensuring that water always enters and exits the body . On the back of the body of the anodonta, the mantle forms two tubes or siphons . The upper one is smooth-walled and is called the excretory or cloacal siphon. Through it , water

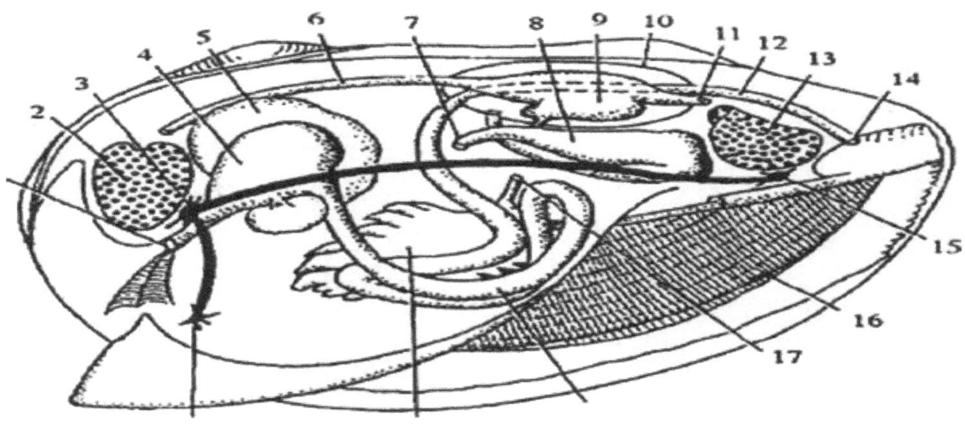

29- Fig. Structure of bivalve mollusks scheme.

l-mouth, 2-anterior obturator muscle, 3-cerebropleural ganglion, 4-stomach, 5-liver, 6-anterior aorta, 7- external renal aperture, 8-kidney opening into the precordium, 9-heart, 10-pericardium, 11-posterior aorta, 12-posterior intestine, 13-posterior obturator muscle, 14-anal orifice, 15-visceral parietal ganglion, 16-

gills, 17-gonadal aperture , 18- midgut, 19-gonadal gland, 20-pedal ganglion.

The respiratory organs consist of right and left gill plates, which are symmetrically arranged relative to each other . Accordingly , bivalves are also called plate gills. Each gill plate is double-layered , forming an inner and outer membrane. does.

Water entering through the Jabra siphon fills the mantle cavity, then washes the Jabra plates, passes into the Jabra cavity, and exits through the discharge siphon.

Gas exchange occurs in the gills, taking in oxygen dissolved in the water and releasing carbon dioxide.

The circulatory system of anodonta is open, with the heart located within the pericardial sac (pericardial cavity), a remnant of the secondary body cavity (coelom) on the dorsal side of the body.

The heart consists of two chambers and one ventricle. The aorta branches off the ventricles anteriorly and posteriorly . Blood passes from the aorta to the arteries. It is pumped throughout the body through capillaries, while the carbon dioxide-rich blood passes through the lacunae and enters the body through veins , where it is oxidized and carried to the heart chambers. is coming.

From there, it passes into the ventricle of the heart and spreads back to the body through the aorta.

Identify the anterior and posterior sides of the body of the anodonta . Draw a picture of the top view of the shell . Draw.

1. If possible, observe a live anaconda in an aquarium . Pay attention to the movement of the muscular legs . Observe the entry and exit of water from the siphons . To do this, drip some colored solution (dew, carmine) onto the back of the anaconda in the aquarium . Pay attention to the colored solution entering through the inlet siphon and exiting through the outlet siphon give.

2. To study the internal structure of the anodonta, hot water is poured between the shells . Then, insert a surgical knife between the shells of the anodonta and cut the anterior and posterior obturator muscles in the ligamentous sheath. As a result, the shells open. Place the split anodonta in a preparation bath and pour water over it until the body is submerged in water. Then, with a pair of scissors , lift one

edge of the mantle membrane and the mantle cavity and gill plates underneath are visible . Observe the inlet and outlet siphons at the end of the mantle membrane . To study the intestines, heart, and other organelles of the anodonta, the body is divided in two using a scalpel starting from the base of the leg . Picture of the internal structure of the anodonta Draw.

Assignments on the topic .

1. Draw a picture of the shell of an anodonta in your notebook . 2. one per minute how much in the distance pushed define.

3. Draw a picture of what you see in the internal structure of anodonta in your notebook. Draw.

Control questions:

1. The external structure of the larynx ?
2. The living conditions of the anaconda and spread?
3. What organs are in the head of the mantle of the eel? located?
4. What is the digestive system of a frog like? structured?

13 -Laboratory Exercise.

Topic:Chelicerata, Arachnids The external and internal structure of a spider, a representative of the class (Arachnida) .

Phylum: Arthropoda - Arthropoda Class: Arachnida - Arachnida Order: Spiders - Araneina

Representative: Spider spider - Arachnius diadamatus Common solpug - Galeodes araneoides

Purpose of the work : To consolidate knowledge on the topic using posters and micropreparations.

Required equipment:

Fixed-bodied spider, mouthparts, legs and spider

Microscopy prepared from saliva , microscope, table and hand magnifier, straightener needle.

Theoretical part: The spider is useful and plays a significant role in destroying pests in agriculture. The head has 8 eyes on the front of the thorax, the spider has 6 pairs of legs, one pair of which is a large strong chelicera (jaw). The last segment of the chelicera has a passage for the venom gland. Two pairs of legs have 6 joints and are called pedipalps. Three pairs of spider saliva are located on the back of the abdomen. The anal opening is located next to the salivary gland.

In spiders, the main joint of the chelicerae and pedipalps acts as a mouth organ . Spiders kill their prey and secrete saliva into its body . Under the influence of saliva, the internal tissues of their prey break down and become liquid. After that, they suck up the liquid food. The food of the spider is digested outside the intestine will be.

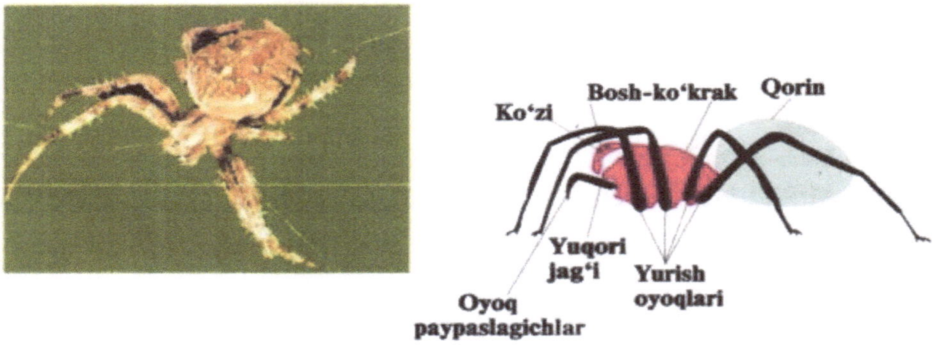

Fig. Exterior of a hermit spider structure.

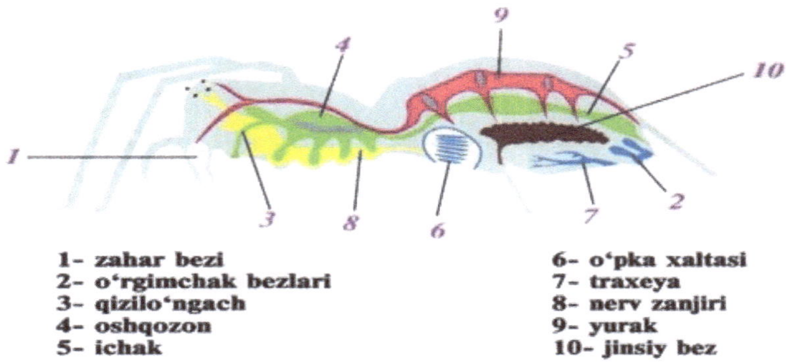

31- Fig. The interior of a hermit spider structure.

Arachnids are unisexual, with well-developed sexual dimorphism. Their gonads are paired, but often the glands are partially fused, forming an odd-numbered organ. The next two segments are located freely in the middle of the cephalothorax, the abdomen consists of 10 segments.

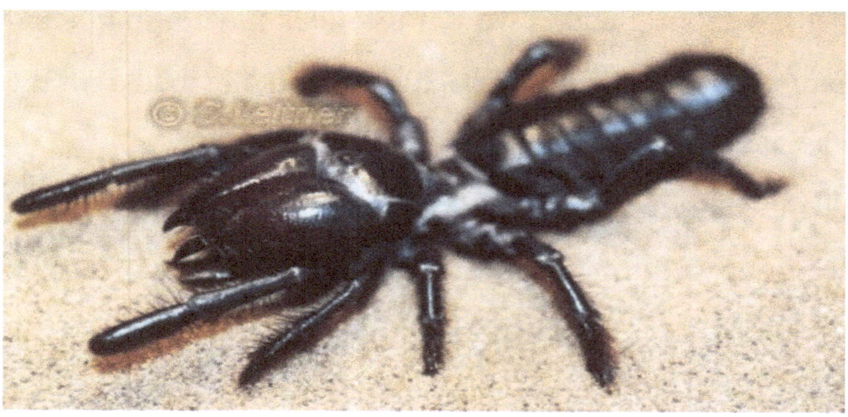

Fig. Black -headed Caspian left-handed

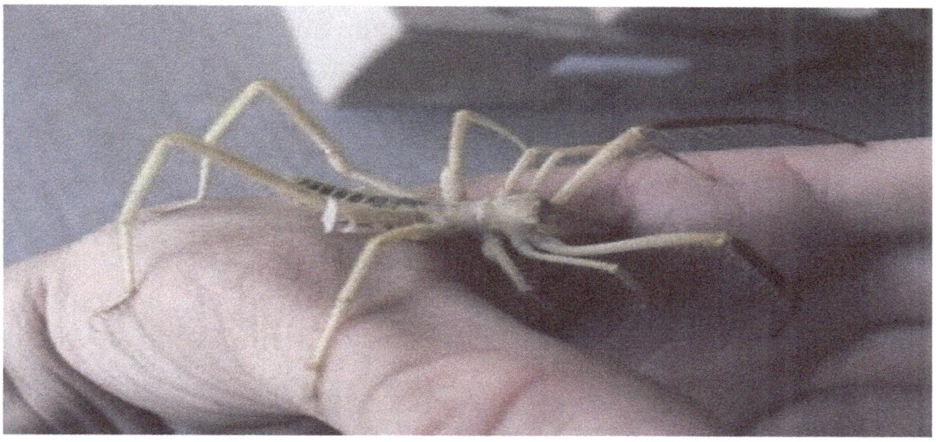

33- Fig. Yellowing left-handed

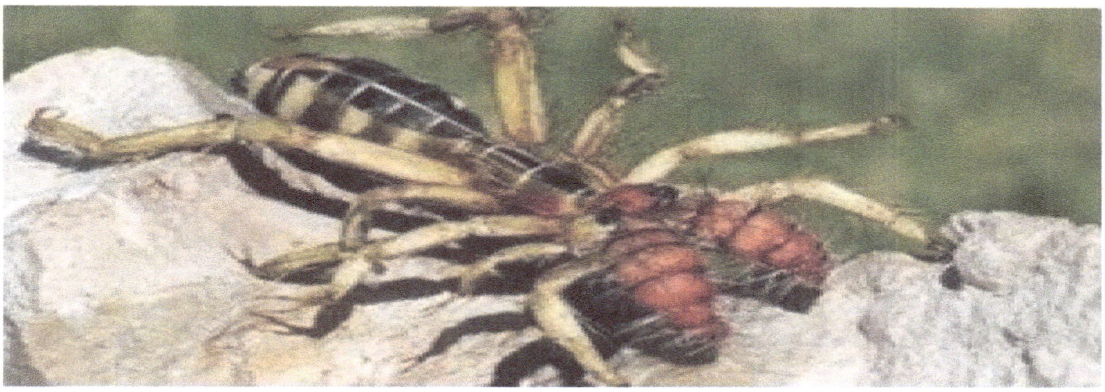

34- Fig. Solpugs types.

The first segment of the cephalothorax contains chelicerae , which are adapted for capturing and killing prey. The pedipalps on the second segment of the cephalothorax look like walking legs. However, they are covered with barbed hairs, which act as

Solpugs are widespread in warm countries. They are predatory arachnids found in the Crimea, the Caucasus, Kazakhstan and Central Asia. They do not have poison-producing glands , but the remains of food (protein substances) in their chelicerae can decompose and turn into poison. Solpugs bite, pierce the skin of people in order to defend themselves (when they try to touch them with their hands) , and are contaminated chelicerae with mechanic in a way to the wound infection infection possible.

Work order:

1. To study the external structure of a spider, place the fixed spider in a watch glass using tweezers and examine its structure using a hand magnifying glass. Find the eyes on the head and the fluid points on one side of the abdomen. Observe the abdomen using a hand magnifying glass and pay attention to their placement on the abdomen. give.

2. the fixed salpugs in a petri dish and observe them using a hand magnifying glass. Find its cephalothorax and abdomen. Pay attention to the segmentation of its body and the chelicerae . Draw a picture of the external structure of a salpug Draw.

Assignments on the topic.

1. Draw the external structure of a spider and a wasp in your notebook. 2. Count the legs of the spiders and identify their functions and draw them in your notebook.

Control questions:

1. What is the structure of a spider ? 2. What is the habitat of a spider? conditions? 3. How many walking legs does a solpug have and how are they structured?

14- Laboratory Exercise

Subject: Subphylum Tracheata, Large class Hexapoda or Insecta, Class Insecta- Ectognatha, Family of water striders - black water strider, The external structure of a locust, a representative of the order of the Orthoptera, and a May beetle, a representative of the order of the Beetles . Phylum: Arthropoda - Arthropoda Class: Insecta - Insecta Category: Cockroaches - BlattoideaRepresentative: Black cockroach - Blatta vrientalis

Purpose of the work:

To develop students' ability to work independently by conducting experiments on live aquatic animals.

Required equipment: live scads (female and male), chloroform, baths, plates showing the external structure of the scad , preparation tubes, entomological tweezers, hand-held magnifying glasses, binoculars, small sharp-tipped scissors, item bottles, surgery knives, white cardboard of paper the beads.

Theoretical part:

Cockroaches are common in houses (apartments), barns, bakeries , kitchens and other places where food is available for them. Their cylindrical body is 2-3 cm long, flattened from the shoulders to the abdomen . The difference between the sexes (sexual dimorphism) is clearly expressed. The body of females is wider than that of males, and their wings are undeveloped (rudimentary). .

currently widespread Central Asian ladybug (Shelgortella tartara) has yellow dots on the last thoracic and first abdominal segments . The wings of the males of this ladybug are much longer than their bodies, and by these signs they are distinguished from the black ladybug (Vlatta orientalis). Like all other insects , the ladybug's body consists of three sections: the head, thorax, and abdomen , covered with a chitinous shell. The head (cephalon) is connected to the body by a thin ridge on the neck . It is formed by the fusion of 5 segments . The ladybug's head is triangular in shape, covered with a thick chitinous shell and turned into a cephalon. Its lower part is the mouth, and the upper part is the forehead. On both sides of the head are a pair of antennae consisting of fine, fine hairs . They perform the functions of smell (chemoreceptors) and touch . Seeing a pair of complex faceted eyes at the base of the whiskers possible.

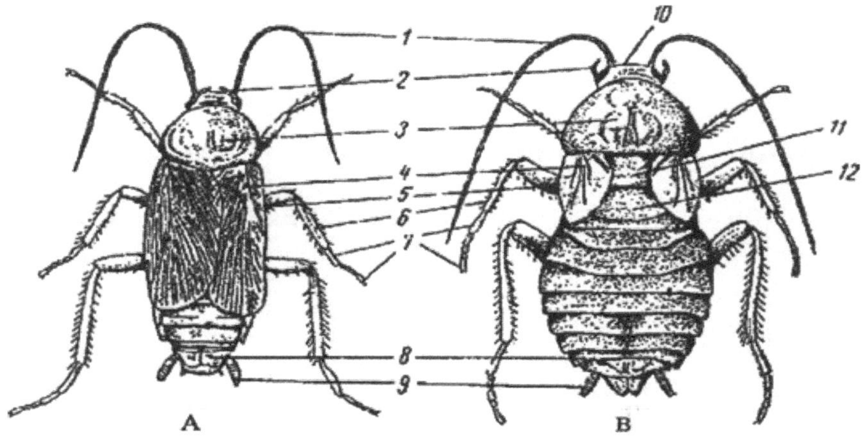

36. External appearance of a male water strider (Periplaneta americana) structure .

External structure of a male (A) and female (B) water strider.

1 - whiskers, 2 - mandibles, 3 - anterior thoracic joint, 4 - upper wing, 5 - thigh, 6 - lower leg, 7 - paw, 8 - tenth abdominal joint, 9 - scutes, 10 - head, 11 - middle thoracic joint, 12 - **hind thoracic joint.**

The thorax is composed of three segments , each of which independently forms a separate section of the thorax . Accordingly, the thorax is divided into the anterior, middle, and posterior thorax. The thorax of water striders, and in general of all insects, is a locomotor body section. Because this section contains three pairs of legs and two pairs (except for dipterans) of wings located.

Males of water voles have well-developed wings, but they are not adapted for flight . Females have short and very short wings . The front pair of wings is attached to the middle thorax , forming a thick and hard wing covert . The second pair of wings is much thinner. will be.

hexapods (Nexopods) because they have three pairs of walking legs in their thorax . All their legs are the same. The first pair of legs (the front legs) are attached to the anterior thorax, the second pair to the middle thorax, and the third pair to the posterior thorax. The legs consist of five main joints - the rump, the rump, the thigh, the shin, and the paw (palm). The posterior part of the body ends with a pair of claws . The legs of water striders are adapted for running. Their claws are relatively long and slightly flattened. The legs of this type have special devices on their paws . Under the claws are or ether, cotton, sharp-pointed scissors, thin-pointed tweezers, entomological tweezers, plates depicting the internal structure of the spore, microscope slides, and coverslips.

Theoretical part: Study the structure of the internal organ system of the saurian the most

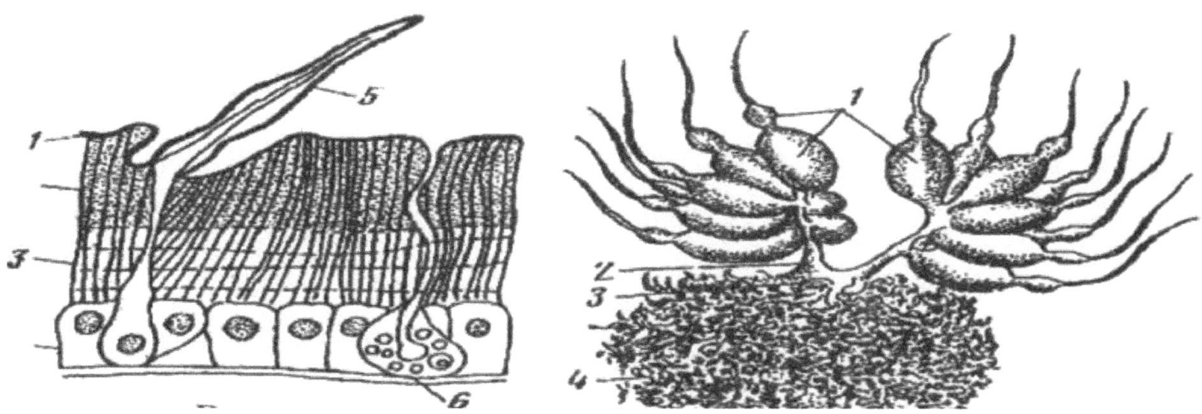

avvalo uning qon aylanish organlaridan boshlash maqsadga muvofiqdir, chunki

The heart of the swarovski crystal is located on the inner surface of the cut shoulder blade.

will be .

The heart is a long tube-shaped organ that consists of 13 chambers. Each chamber has 1 salivary gland reservoir , 2. salivary gland , 3 jigildian, 4 muscular stomach, 5. midgut, Malpighian tubules, 7. hindgut, 8. 9. trachea, 10. abdominal nerve chain, 11. testicles, 1 2 gonads, 13. heart, 14. brain, 15. sympathetic nervous system, 16. pyloric (caecal) appendages

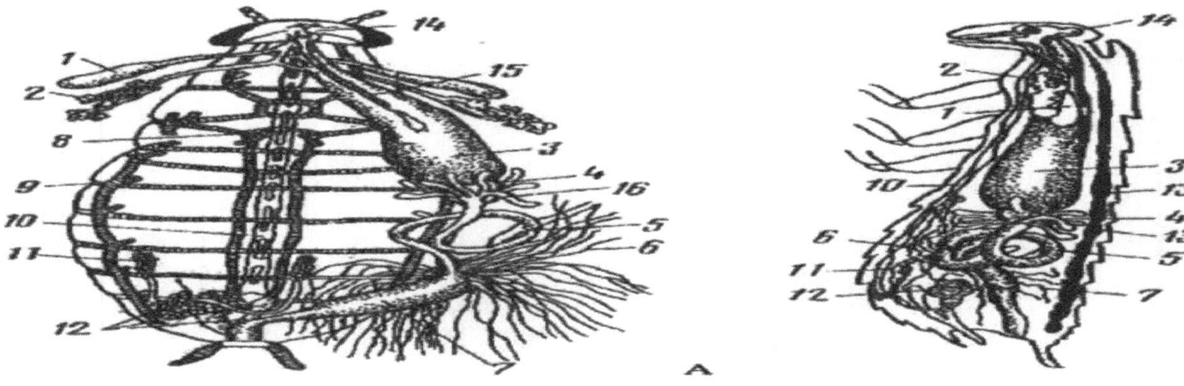

37. Internal structure of the water tank

Black watering structure . A . inside structure back and side view :

A pair of salivary glands open. The posterior part of these glands expands to form a reservoir for collecting saliva . The saliva serves to moisten solid food. The pharynx of the scrotum turns into a rather short esophagus. The esophagus expands like a sac to form the gizzard. After it is located the muscular stomach. With the help of chitinous "teeth" in its inner wall, food is thoroughly ground . The pharynx , esophagus, gizzard, and muscular stomach form the anterior part of the intestine. The posterior part of the muscular stomach is the cardia turned into a valve .

passes food into the midgut and prevents it from moving in the opposite direction. The midgut is a thin cylindrical tube . At its anterior beginning there are 8 pylar glands. They, like the midgut, perform the function of absorbing food. The hindgut (large intestine) consists of two sections, the anterior part of which is thin, and the posterior part is thickened, which opens to the outside through the anal opening. In the hindgut , the water contained in the digested food is reabsorbed again , and the undigested food residues are collected in the posterior (rectal) section of the hindgut and excreted.

The inner surface of the foregut and hindgut of insects, including the cuticle, is covered with cuticle. covered.

excretory system of the midgut consists of long, white, filamentous Malpighian tubules that join at the junction of the midgut and hindgut . The free ends of these tubules are closed, but their interior opens into the pit and hindgut. In addition to the excretory organs , fat bodies can also be found. The cells of the fat bodies also secrete substances that need to be excreted from the body cavity of the midgut and are formed during the process of metabolism . However, they are not excreted, but are accumulated and stored there until the end of the insect's life. At the same time, fat bodies serve as a necessary nutrient for the insect's diet . does.

The central nervous system of the saurian consists of the supralaryngeal and infralaryngeal ganglia, and the ventral nerve cord. The supralaryngeal ganglia, or forebrain, consists of three sections. The anterior section is the protacerebrum, the middle section is the deutacerebrum, and the posterior section is the tritacerebrum.

Water striders are unisexual . In females, the reproductive system consists of a pair of ovaries and oviducts. Each egg consists of eight tubes containing eggs . In addition to these, the female reproductive organs also include a sperm-receiving and an accessory gland . The fluid produced by the accessory gland of the water strider forms

Pour it into water and observe it through binoculars. Note its stringy texture and tiny rings.

1. the head of the water strider to the body , cut off the thin neck with scissors, and observe its head with a magnifying glass . To do this, place the head in a bathtub with an entomological microscope, looking from front to back . In this way, the mouth and gill openings of the water strider are clearly visible.
2. Separate one of the legs of a water strider and place a drop of water in a glass container and observe it using binoculars or a hand-held magnifying glass. Identify and draw its main joints. Draw.
3. Separate each of the three segments that make up the thorax with small, sharp scissors , and examine the second pair of wings using binoculars or a magnifying glass. watch.
4. Separate the abdominal cavity and the male's scrotum from the abdomen of the scrotum , item in the bottle one drop to the water pour and binocular using follow
5. To study the internal organs of the saurac, it is necessary to open it. To do this

, hold the saurac with the abdomen down and the head towards the anterior end . Then, with thin scissors , cut the junction of the tergites and sternites on the side from the posterior end of the saurac's body to the anterior thorax . Turn the head of the saurac towards you and cut the left end in the same way as described above . Connect the lateral sections with a transverse cut from the anterior thorax . Then , place the saurac in a bath and firmly pinch the head and posterior end of the abdomen with forceps . Hold the last segment of the tergite with forceps , wait a while and cut the muscles and trachea holding it with scissors. Separate the tergite , fix it with its inner surface facing up in the bath with forceps and remove the multi-chambered heart of the saurac. watch.

6. around the intestine of the saurian through a hand magnifying glass . Then, separate some of the fat bodies with forceps , place them in a drop of water in a glass slide, cover with a coverslip, and examine them through the small and then the large objectives of the microscope. watch.

7. To study the digestive system, cut off the posterior end of the hindgut with scissors and hold it with forceps, wait a moment, then cut off the anterior part of the intestine , and then observe the division of the intestinal tube into sections using a hand magnifying glass . Note the blind spots at the beginning of the midgut. give.

10. Remove the Malpighian worms from the intestine, place them in a drop of water in a glass slide, and observe them through a small microscope objective or binoculars.

11. Observe the reproductive system through a hand magnifying glass and determine the sex of the frog.

12.0 the digestive and reproductive systems and observe the abdominal nerve cord above them using a hand magnifying glass. Draw a picture of the structure of the internal organs of the saurian, showing the shoulder and side views. Draw.

Assignments on the topic .

The interior of the water tank structure :

a) Blood rotation

b) Digestion to do

c) Genitourinary system

d) Draw a diagram of the structure of the nervous system in your notebook.

Control questions:

1. The size and external structure of the water tank how?
2. What is the nervous system of a water strider ? structured?

15 -Laboratory exercise.

Topic: The development of insects that undergo incomplete metamorphosis - grasshoppers, grasshoppers, dragonflies and wasps, and insects that undergo complete metamorphosis - mulberry silkworms and Colorado potato beetles

The of the work. The postembryonic (development after hatching from the egg) period of development of insects occurs through metamorphosis, that is, transformation. Metamorphosis is observed with incomplete development and complete development.

Insects that undergo incomplete metamorphosis include: damselflies, moths (semi-hard-winged), ornithopods, dragonflies, lice, damselflies, bedbugs, and hymenoptera. The larvae that hatch from their eggs are very similar to adult insects, differing from adult insects in their small bodies, underdeveloped wings, and underdeveloped reproductive organs. does.

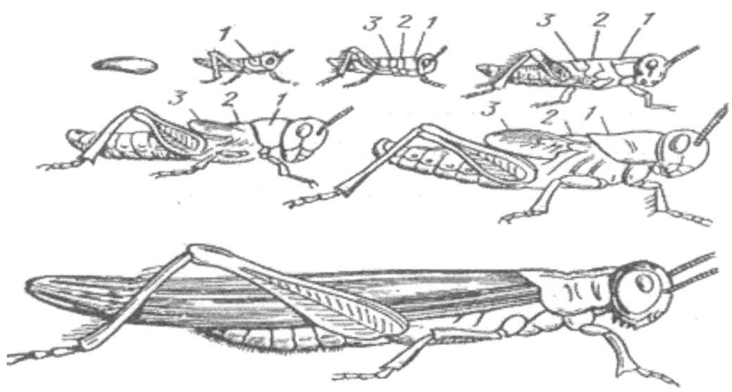

Fig. Grasshopper through premature metamorphosis development.

1,2,3-thoracic joints; first from the left in the top row - egg, in the first and second rows from the top - larvae of different ages, below - adult

A small insect.

The differences between the larva and the imago gradually disappear as a result of a series of molts after the period of their transition from one age to the next. The larvae molt 4-5 times, and then reach sexual maturity (imago). For example, the development of grasshoppers occurs in this order. In insects that develop incompletely, there is no pupation period.

Insects that undergo complete metamorphosis include beetles (hard-winged), butterflies, fleas, diptera, hymenoptera, tetrapods, and a group of other insects. The larvae (worms) that hatch from the eggs of these insects are completely different from the adults (imagos).

These larvae have completely undeveloped wings and only have organs specific to the larval stage. An example of this is the mulberry silkworm. The worm's mouthparts are of a gnawing type, while in butterflies they are of a sucking type.

In addition, the butterfly caterpillar has several pairs of "flying" legs on its abdomen. These false legs are not divided into joints. Butterfly caterpillars also shed their skin five times during their development and enter the pupal stage. pupa

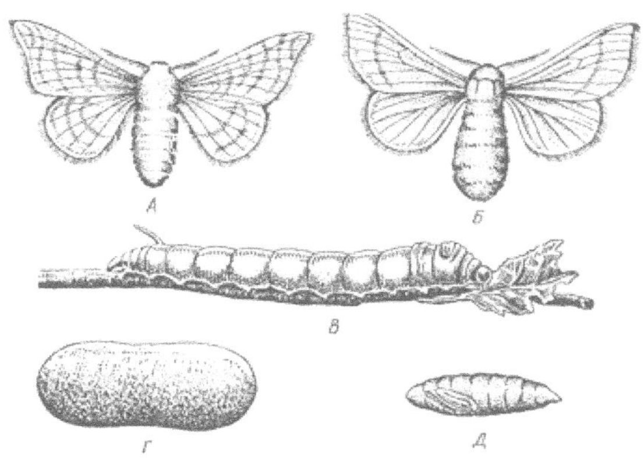

38- Fig. Complete metamorphosis of the mulberry silkworm development.
A-male butterfly, B-female butterfly, V-worm, G-cocoon, D-sponge removed from the cocoon.

It is considered a period of quiet development, during which the pupa develops organs typical of adult butterflies.

Work execution. Place the larvae of different ages of grasshoppers in a Petri dish and, using a hand magnifying glass, pay attention to the structure of the larvae, i.e. wings, legs and other organs. Observe the wings of the imago stage. Do the same with the mulberry silkworm.

Assignments on the topic.

1. Picture the development of a grasshopper Draw.

2. Diagram showing the development of the larva, pupa, cocoon , and butterfly of the mulberry silkworm. draw

Control questions:

1. Insects increase.
2. Insect larvae and their biological role. 3. Fully developed insects.

4. Insects that develop incompletely.

Main literature used.

1. Mavlonov O., Khurramov Sh., Eshova Kh. Invertebrate zoology. Textbook for undergraduate students of higher education institutions specializing in biology. National Encyclopedia of Uzbekistan State Scientific Publishing House. Tashkent 2006.

2. Mavlonov O., Saparov K., Toshmanov N. ZOOLOGY (invertebrates). Biology teaching methodology textbook for undergraduate students. Sano-Standard Publishing House. Tashkent-2018

3. Dadaev S., Saparov K. Laboratory exercises on the subject of invertebrate zoology. A textbook for students of the bachelor's degree program 5110400- Biology Teaching Methods of Higher Pedagogical Universities. Tashkent. Navruz Publishing House. 2020.

4 Dadaev S., Practical application of the subject of invertebrate zoology exercises. Textbook for undergraduate biology students of higher educational institutions. Tashkent. Navruz Publishing House. 2020.

5.Dadaev S. Practical exercises in vertebrate zoology. Textbook. – Tashkent: Bookmany print, 2022. – 346 p. Sharova IX Zoology of invertebrates. Textbook for students of biology. VUZov. M., VLADOS, 2002.

6 Konstantinov VM, Naumov SP, Shatalova SP. Zoologiya pozvonochnyx:Uchebnikdlyastud.uchrejdeniyvyssh.ped. prof. education M.: Izdateliki Center

9 789369 085088

Printed at Repro India Ltd.